Atlas of
AMPLITUDE-INTEGRATED
EEGs in the NEWBORN

Atlas of
AMPLITUDE-INTEGRATED EEGs in the NEWBORN
Second Edition

Lena Hellström-Westas
Department of Women's and Children's Health, Uppsala University,
Uppsala, Sweden

Linda S de Vries
Department of Neonatology, Wilhelmina Children's Hospital
UMC Utrecht, The Netherlands

Ingmar Rosén
Division of Clinical Neurophysiology
Department of Clinical Science
Lund University
Lund, Sweden

Foreword by Terrie Inder

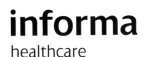

informa
healthcare

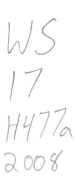

© 2008 Informa UK Ltd

First edition published in the United Kingdom in 2003

Second edition published in the United Kingdom in 2008 by Informa Healthcare, Telephone House, 69–77 Paul Street, London, EC2A 4LQ. Informa Healthcare is a trading division of Informa UK Ltd. Registered Office: 37/41 Mortimer Street, London W1T 3JH. Registered in England and Wales number 1072954

Tel: +44 (0)20 7017 5000
Fax: +44 (0)20 7017 6699
Website: www.informahealthcare.com

A CIP record for this book is available from the British Library.

Library of Congress Cataloging-in-Publication Data

Data available on application

ISBN-10: 1 84184 649 X
ISBN-13: 978 1 84184 649 1

Distributed in North and South America by
Taylor & Francis
6000 Broken Sound Parkway, NW, (Suite 300)
Boca Raton, FL 33487, USA

Within Continental USA
Tel: 1 (800) 272 7737; Fax: 1 (800) 374 3401
Outside Continental USA
Tel: (561) 994 0555; Fax: (561) 361 6018
Email: orders@crcpress.com

Book orders in the rest of the world
Paul Abrahams
Tel: +44 207 017 4036
Email: bookorders@informa.com

Composition by Exeter Premedia Services Private Ltd., Chennai, India
Printed and bound in India by Replika Press Pvt Ltd

Contents

Foreword – *Terrie Inder*   vii
Preface to the first edition   ix
Preface to the second edition   xi
List of abbreviations   xii

1   Methodology   1

2   The electrocortical background, its normal maturation, classification,
    and effects of medication   17

3   Pitfalls and caveats   43

4   Seizures   57

5   Hypoxia–ischemia   79

6   Focal hemorrhagic and ischemic lesions in the full-term infant   109

7   Hemorrhagic and ischemic lesions in the preterm infant   127

8   Metabolic diseases, brain malformations, and central nervous system
    infections   147

References   177

Index   185

Foreword

It is a great honor and pleasure to provide a Foreword to this second edition of *Atlas of Amplitude-Integrated EEGs in the Newborn* which has been carefully prepared by three superb clinical investigators spanning neonatology, neurology, and neurophysiology.

The field of neonatal neurology has gained an increasing momentum over the last few decades with a greater desire by clinicians to understand the pathway to neurodevelopmental disability that is common in survivors of neonatal intensive care. For the term infant with encephalopathy and/or seizures, identification of the extent of brain injury and/or seizures is clinically challenging. Bedside brain monitoring using limited channels of electroencephalography (EEG) with amplitude integration (aEEG) has been shown to better define brain injury and predict outcome than any other method. In a similar fashion, seizure detection with newer aEEG devices with raw EEG has also been shown to detect over three-quarters of conventionally defined EEG seizures. The advantages of such monitoring include that the EEG equipment is portable, easy to apply, and permits continuous monitoring for both background brain activity and seizures. Thus, although aEEG has been available for 40 years, the clinical neonatal milieu has now recognized the requirement for brain monitoring in the NICU setting with interventions for neuroprotection becoming reality with hypothermia and newer anticonvulsant drugs. In addition, there has been an expansion of the available devices for such monitoring with variable numbers of channels and the combination of raw EEG and aEEG tracing. As a result, clinical use of aEEG devices in the term born encephalopathic infant is expanding, with more than one in five term infants being monitored in the USA alone, a country with a recent history in the utility of these tools.

For the preterm infant, clinical identification of brain injury and seizure activity has also been limited. In addition to injury, normative developmental progression can be followed using EEG, assisting in tracking brain maturation and any disturbance.

Whether for the preterm or the term infant, the single most essential component of the successful use of bedside EEG devices is knowledge and accurate interpretation. Significant advances in this field have occurred since the first edition of this book with the types of technologies, the outputs (raw EEG and aEEG), and the broader clinical scenarios that are being monitored. To this end this book is timely and critical in the progression of this field and its integration into NICU monitoring. Such knowledge and assistance spanning the fundamentals of the original and newer technologies through the nature of EEG and aEEG traces in the major clinical settings is an invaluable guide that no NICU should be without.

Associate Professor Terrie Inder
Washington University
St Louis, Missouri, USA

Preface to the first edition

As we have gained experience with the cerebral function monitor (CFM) over the years, it has given us so much valuable clinical information about our patients that we are convinced that it should be available for all newborn intensive care patients.

The technique was introduced in Lund in 1978 after Ingmar Rosén had visited Pamela Prior in London to discuss a method for experimental EEG monitoring. At that time there were several publications on the use of the CFM in adults. Ingmar Rosén, together with Nils Svenningsen, felt that there was a need for more intensive monitoring of brain function in their very vulnerable newborn babies and they were encouraged to try using the monitor. A few years later Lena Hellström-Westas, with the assistance of Ingmar Rosén and Nils Svenningsen, started to evaluate the method in the neonatal intensive care unit (NICU). Linda de Vries visited Lund in 1992 to learn to use the CFM and to interpret the recordings. At that time there were four CFM machines in Lund. Within a few years Utrecht had six machines.

At that stage we had no plans to write an atlas of CFM monitoring together. However, with the increasing use of the CFM all over the world, particularly for the prognosis of asphyxia in the term infant and for selection for intervention studies on, for example, hypothermia for perinatal asphyxia, it has become clear that there is a need for a reference atlas. We also wanted to have an opportunity to give examples of the use of the CFM in other clinical situations.

We planned to write the Atlas of Amplitude-Integrated EEGs in the Newborn together with Nils Svenningsen. Sadly, he died suddenly before we could start the work. He was and is a great inspiration to us and we are dedicating this Atlas to his memory.

We are grateful to the many people who have worked on developing and promoting the use of the CFM. First, we want to thank Pamela Prior for introducing the method to us and for generously sharing her experience of the CFM with us. We also want to thank Douglas Maynard for his discussions on CFM development and on the Cerebral Function Analysing Monitor (CFAM). We thank Marianne Thoresen who, together with Douglas Maynard, contributed a nice CFAM example. We are also grateful for stimulating CFM discussions with Klara Thiringer, Eva Thornberg, Gorm Greisen and Denis Azzopardi and for all the input we have received from CFM sessions at the European Neonatal Brain Club. In order to stress the utility of a method rather than a commercially available machine, we have applied Gorm Greisen's term 'amplitude-integrated EEG' (aEEG) throughout the Atlas.

Introducing the CFM into our NICUs was easy and all the neonatologists quickly learned to interpret the traces. We would like to thank Floris Groenendaal, Paula Eken, Karin Rademaker, Kristina Thorngren-Jerneck, Helena Klette and, especially, Mona Toet all of whom have contributed to publications that are quoted in the Atlas. We are also grateful to Kees van Huffelen who helped to compare the CFM and the standard EEG. We are happy for and much appreciate all technical assistance and support that we received from May Vitestam, Elin Persson, Paul Mikkelsen and Lars-Johan Ahnlide. Much of this work could not have been done without the enthusiastic support of all the nurses in our units who quickly learned how to attach the monitor to a baby, obtain a good recording and to appreciate the significance of the traces. Thanks go especially to Marianne Buikema and Joke Zoet who were involved in producing a wonderful teaching CD Rom.

Finally, we hope that many babies will benefit from this Atlas and that the reader will find it a practical reference, a good learning experience and have as much fun going through it as we had putting it together.

Lena Hellström-Westas
Linda S de Vries
Ingmar Rosén

Preface to the second edition

We are very pleased to present this revised second edition of *Atlas of Amplitude-Integrated EEGs in the Newborn*. The first edition was published in 2003. Since then the aEEG has been increasingly used in many neonatal intensive care units and the number of publications evaluating various aspects of the aEEG is growing almost exponentially. Recently, the first meta-analysis, evaluating the aEEG for prediction of outcome in term asphyxiated infants, was published. The authors concluded that the aEEG is useful for prediction of outcome and recommended it to be a part of the initial evaluation of all infants after perinatal asphyxia.

The idea behind the predecessor of the aEEG, the Cerebral Function Monitor, which was created and explored by Maynard, Prior, and Scott back in the 1960s, was to design a stable and simple monitor that could be used by the intensive-care staff for evaluation of brain function. With the introduction of new digital aEEG monitors, new possibilities for advanced monitoring of newborn infants have become possible. The gap between the aEEG and the standard EEG is closing, since several of the new monitors can also record aEEG from a variable number of channels as well as a full EEG. Within the near future, other EEG trends than the aEEG will be explored and evaluated.

We are very grateful to several people who contributed with their knowledge and time to create this Atlas: Marianne Thoresen, Frances Cowan, Denis Azzopardi, Sampsa Vanhatalo, Katarina Strand-Brodd, Graham McBain, Heidar Einarsson, Gardar Thorvardson, Ted Weiler, and Damon Lees.

We would also especially like to thank: the late Nils Svenningsen, who was extremely important for the initial introduction of aEEG in the neonatal intensive care unit; Lars-Johan Ahnlide, who created the first digital aEEG/EEG monitor by 'reversed engineering' in the late 1990s, and who continues to work with aEEG with never-failing enthusiasm; Mona Toet, who created an aEEG database in Utrecht, which helped us to select the best case histories of all those collected since 1992; Kees van Huffelen, with his vast neurophysiologic expertise has been most supportive and contributed to improve the technique; Gorm Greisen, Linda van Rooij, Elisabeth Norman, David Ley, Damjan Osredkar, Floris Groenendaal, and Sverre Wikström for good collaboration in research on aEEG.

Much of this work could not have been done without the enthusiastic support of all the nurses and EEG technicians who quickly learned how to attach the monitor to a baby, obtain a good recording, and to appreciate the significance of the traces. Our special thanks go to Joke Zoet, Ann-Cathrine Berg, Bodil Persson, Suze van Kogelenberg-Wickel, and Ben Nieuwenstein.

Finally, we hope that many babies will benefit from this Atlas and that the reader will find it a practical reference, a good learning experience, and enjoy it as much as we did putting it together.

Lena Hellström-Westas
Linda S de Vries
Ingmar Rosén

List of abbreviations

AC	Alternate current		Hb	Hemoglobin
aEEG	Amplitude-integrated EEG		HFV	High-frequency ventilation
AS	Active sleep		HIE	Hypoxic–ischemic encephalopathy
BE	Base excess		IBI	Interburst interval
BF	Burst frequency		ICH	Intracranial hemorrhage
BS	Burst suppression		ICU	Intensive care unit
BW	Birthweight		ip	Intraperitoneal
CFAM	Cerebral function analyzing monitor		iv	Intravenous
CFM	Cerebral function monitor		Lido	Lidocaine
CNV	Continuous normal voltage aEEG in full-term infant		Mida	Midazolam
			MRI	Magnetic resonance imaging
CS	Cesarean section		NEC	Necrotizing enterocolitis
CSA	Compressed spectral array		NICU	Neonatal intensive care unit
CSF	Cerebrospinal fluid		NIRS	Near-infrared spectroscopy
CTG	Cardio tocography		PCA	Postconceptional age
DC	Direct current		Phenob	Phenobarbitone
DNV	Discontinuous normal voltage aEEG in full-term infant		Pheny	Phenytoin
			PLED	Periodic lateralized discharge
DQ	Developmental quotient		PROM	Premature rupture of membranes
DSA	Density spectral array		PRSW	Positive rolandic sharp wave
DWI	Diffusion weighted imaging		PVL	Periventricular leukomalacia
ECG	Electrocardiography		PWMI	Periventricular white matter injury
ECMO	Extracorporeal membrane oxygenation		RDS	Respiratory distress syndrome
			REM	Rapid eye movement
EEG	Electroencephalography		QS	Quiet sleep
FFT	Fast Fourier transformation		SAT	Spontaneous activity transients
FT	Flat trace (EEG/aEEG)		SEF	Spectral edge frequency
FTOE	Fractional cerebral tissue oxygen extraction		SEP	Sensory evoked potential
			SWC	Sleep–wake cycling
GA	Gestational age		US	Ultrasound
GMH-IVH	Germinal matrix-intraventricular hemorrhage		W	Wakefulness
			WMD	White matter damage

1

Methodology

Continuous electroencephalographic (EEG) monitoring is a relatively new modality in adult as well as in pediatric and neonatal intensive care units. Whereas a number of physiologic parameters such as electrocardiogram (ECG), heart rate, oxygen saturation, blood pressure, and temperature have long since been integrated into intensive care unit (ICU) monitoring systems, monitoring of the EEG, which directly reflects the functional state of the brain, has been used less commonly. There are probably a number of reasons for this:

(1) The brain-generated EEG signal is of low amplitude, and easily contaminated by artifacts of both biologic and non-biologic origin. Interpretation of the EEG requires extensive training that includes good knowledge about sources of artifacts. Furthermore, due consideration has to be given to a number of factors such as level of wakefulness and administered medications, and in neonatal patients also to gestational age and postconceptional age.

(2) A major disadvantage with intermittently recorded neonatal conventional EEGs is the difficulty, for the attending clinician as well as for the EEG specialist, to discriminate emerging trends of development of the electrocerebral activity over hours and days, which directly reflects clinically relevant pathophysiologic processes.

(3) Even with the development of new electrode caps, the intensive care situation does not usually permit surveillance and maintenance of impedances and positions of multiple EEG recording electrodes on the scalp for any length of time exceeding a few hours.

In order to have a clinical impact on medical decisions and later outcome, monitoring of the electrocortical activity should be continuous, with a simple recording set-up and a small number of recording electrodes.

NEURONAL BASIS FOR EEG

Individual thalamocortical relay cells, and cells in the thalamic reticular nucleus, as well as cortical pyramidal cells each have recurrent action potential firing properties.[1] The activity within groups of thalamocortical neurons is synchronized by recurrent connections between thalamocortical relay cells and the surrounding reticular thalamic nucleus, and also between the thalamus and the cortex (see Figure 1.1a). Furthermore, recurrent connections within the cortex itself generate high frequency EEG components during active wakefulness and mental processes. During arousal, cholinergic (and noradrenergic) afferents from the brainstem exert an excitatory depolarizing effect on thalamocortical and cortical cells and inhibit the reticular thalamic cells. The net result of arousal is a reduction of synchronous low frequency activity, and an increase of asynchronous high frequency activity, as illustrated in Figure 1.1b.

During fetal development, and also including the first period of life in the extremely preterm infant, a transient fetal subplate zone is situated between the white matter and the cortical plate. The fetal subplate zone is the origin of thalamocortical and corticocortical afferents and probably contributes to EEG activity both directly and indirectly via its cortical connections.[2] The subplate zone is of particular interest for the mechanisms underlying the spontaneous activity transients (SATs), which are dominated by very low frequency waves with higher frequency components superimposed, a predominant feature of the early preterm EEG.[3–5]

CFM AND aEEG

Maynard constructed the original cerebral function monitor (CFM) in the late 1960s in response to clinical needs for continuous EEG monitoring in adult intensive care.[6] The method's clinical applications were developed by Prior, mainly in adult patients during anesthesia and in intensive care, e.g. after cardiac arrest, during status epilepticus, and after heart surgery.[7,8] Lectromed (Letchworth, UK) and Criticon (Florida, USA) produced some of the first versions of the CFM. The technique and major clinical applications of the CFM are summarized in the book *Monitoring Cerebral Function: Long Term Monitoring of EEG and Evoked Potentials* by PF Prior and DE Maynard,[9] to which the reader is referred for details. In the present Atlas we have used the term aEEG to denote a method for electrocortical monitoring rather than a specific machine.

The EEG signal for the aEEG is recorded from one channel (optional two channels) with two symmetric parietal electrodes (or four symmetric frontoparietal electrodes derived into two frontoparietal recording channels). The recommended positions of the recording electrodes when using a one or two channel recording are shown in Figure 1.2. It is important to keep the recommended interelectrode distances in order not to alter the amplitude of the recorded EEG signal. The electrodes shown are thin subdermal needles, which in our experience produce a stable and artifact-free recording for hours and even days. The very thin needle electrodes produce no, or very little, discomfort when placed in hairy parts of the skull. However, any conventional EEG electrodes, disk electrodes or disposable stick-on EEG electrodes can be used as alternatives. Hydrogel electrodes are suitable for extremely preterm infants during the first week of life. They can be easily attached after gentle skin preparation with an abrasive cream, e.g. Nuprep® (DO Weaver & Co, Aurora, USA). With surface electrodes it is usually more difficult to get acceptable input impedances in term infants, although some systems work well after training. Furthermore, development of new electrodes is also in progress.

SIGNAL PROCESSING IN THE aEEG

When creating the aEEG, the EEG signal is first amplified and passed through an asymmetric band-pass filter which strongly attenuates activity below 2 Hz and above 15 Hz. This filtering will minimize artifacts from sweating, movements, muscle activity, ECG, and electrical interference (see Figure 1.3). Notably, with a high-pass filter set at 2 Hz a significant part of the low frequency components of the neonatal EEG signal is attenuated. Between 2 and 15 Hz, the filter shape compensates for the fact that the electric energy of the non-rhythmic components of the EEG signal tends to decrease with increasing frequency (approximately 12 dB/decade). The aEEG processing also includes semilogarithmic amplitude compression (linear display 0–10 µV; logarithmic display 10–100 µV), rectifying, smoothing with a time constant of 0.5 s, and time compression.

In the first CFM the signal was written out on slow paper speed, 6 cm/h or 30 cm/h (CFM Multitrace 2 paper speed 1 mm/min to 100 mm/min). The upper and lower borders of the output trace reflect variations in maximum and minimum EEG amplitudes, respectively, as shown in Figures 1.4a and b. As a result of the time constant of the aEEG display, the lower border of the aEEG trace is determined by both the amplitude and spacing of peaks in the EEG. In the presence of repeated discontinuities (interburst interval (IBI) = 1–5 s), the position of the lower border is greatly affected by the interburst interval (see Figure 1.4c). The semilogarithmic output enhances the sensitivity for detection of changes in background activity of very low (<5 µV) amplitudes. The information in the aEEG trace can be enhanced by modifying the gray scale so that the darkness of a particular spot is determined by the length of time spent at that spot. This feature is helpful in defining the lower border of the trace and changes caused by ictal periods (Figure 1.5).

In the original CFM, electrode impedance was recorded simultaneously and displayed on a second channel and also included an overload detection function (at >800 µV peak-to-peak). Extracerebral sources of signals below this level, but falling within the frequency window of the EEG recorder, will add to the displayed aEEG with a risk of misinterpretation as a result.

This drawback has been substantially alleviated by the recent development of several new EEG/aEEG-monitors based on digital techniques. The new pieces of equipment (Figure 1.6) make it possible to process and store the aEEG together with the original EEG signal. This also enhances the possibility for more reliable online discrimination of artifacts from real EEG signals (Figure 1.7). Also very short duration events (seconds), such as brief epileptic seizures, can now be detected (see Chapter 4). In addition, the original

EEG can also be displayed from stored data post hoc, making it possible to make second opinion evaluations of the recorded data. Some of the new monitors are flexible in terms of number of available recording channels, which is a great advantage for monitoring of status epilepticus also in children after the neonatal period, e.g. in pediatric intensive care. In fact, some of the machines can also be used for recording a full EEG. Due to the major advantages of the simultaneous displays of aEEG and the original EEG signal, we have aimed to illustrate the majority of the cases in this Atlas with recordings by the various new digital equipments.

When the new development of digital equipment started, there was already a substantial amount of worldwide clinical experience accumulated with the old CFM technique. This was also summarized in the first edition of the Atlas. Since the old CFM method had proved to produce clinically useful information, it was considered important to make the performance of the new algorithms for the aEEG calculation as close as possible to the old one, which was done by 'reversed engineering'.[10] It is important to remember that the algorithms used in the different monitors are not identical, although close enough to provide clinically comparable information. Although the original CFM paradigm was developed for use in adult intensive care, it has proved to be useful also in neonatal monitoring.[11-14] However, this technology would probably have been different, if it had been developed de novo for neonatal application. Probably, the ideal EEG trend monitor for neonatal use has yet to be developed.

BASIC aEEG FEATURES OF THE ACUTELY COMPROMISED BRAIN

An acute and critical change in cerebral perfusion or metabolism markedly affects the amplitude and continuity of the EEG signal, whereas more gradual and moderate changes primarily modify the frequency composition of the EEG. During the late recovery phase after a severe acute insult, the EEG also shows more moderate changes, or 'chronic stage abnormalities' (see Figure 1.8).[15] Figure 1.9 shows changes in the CFM aEEG trace with corresponding EEG traces before, during, and at restitution after severe experimental hypoglycemia in a rat.[16] At the onset of the hypoglycemia (trace 2) the amplitude of the EEG signal increases, particularly within the low-frequency EEG components. This causes a moderate increase of the CFM maximum and minimum levels. More profound hypoglycemia results in a discontinuous

burst-suppression (BS) pattern (trace 3), reflecting a functional disconnection of the thalamocortical neuronal circuitry. In the CFM, the minimum border of the trace approaches the zero line, reflecting the isoelectric interburst intervals, whereas the maximum level is maintained, reflecting the high peak-to-peak amplitudes within the intermittent bursts of activity. A period of complete electrocerebral inactivity ensues (trace 4). The recovery of the EEG after glucose infusion is initiated by a brief period of seizure activity with repeated sharp waves (trace 5). In the CFM trace this is seen as an abrupt increase from the zero line. Without the simultaneous original EEG this single brief episode of epileptic activity would not have been recognized from the CFM trace alone. During the subsequent recovery the frequency content of the continuous EEG changes from predominantly low frequency (trace 6) to mixed frequencies (trace 7), accompanied by only minor changes of the CFM trace.

OTHER EEG TRENDS

The digital techniques make it possible to apply new parameters for trend monitoring. Of particular interest for neonatal applications, especially in the very preterm infant and in infants developing or recovering from hypoxic–ischemic insults, are options for direct quantification of the discontinuous EEG activity, e.g. IBI, % suppression, burst frequency (BF), and burst duration (see examples in Figures 1.10a and b). Furthermore, power spectral analysis can also give additional important information on the quality of the electrocortical background in different groups of neonates. Spectral edge frequency (SEF) is calculated as the frequency below which a certain amount (often 80–95%) of the total EEG power resides and has been found to be of relevance in experimental and clinical studies of white matter injury in preterm infants.[17]

More complete displays of the absolute or relative distribution of the EEG frequencies over time are also available (Figure 1.11). The spectral content of the bursts during discontinuous EEG may also turn out to provide clinically useful information. Recent studies show that low-frequency (recorded with a direct current (DC) method) components are predominant in the intermittent SATs of the premature EEG. Recording and monitoring of these in clinical practice will require new developments in terms of electrodes and amplifiers. Automatic seizure detection is a new feature in some of the new EEG monitors that is currently explored. As neonatal seizure patterns are very variable, such a system would probably have to be adjusted individually to each patient in order to obtain an optimal sensitivity and specificity. Future development of EEG monitoring will probably include integrated systems displaying several EEG trends simultaneously, and will also include other physiologic parameters such as arterial blood pressure, oxygen saturation, and cerebral perfusion parameters measured by near infrared spectroscopy (NIRS) (Figure 1.12).

SUMMARY

- Continuous aEEG monitoring offers a possibility to directly monitor the functional state of the brain over hours and days.

- The aEEG/CFM technique was developed to fit into the ICU setting and to present the information in a mode that can be interpreted at bedside. The technique was early introduced also into the neonatal intensive care unit (NICU).

- New digital aEEG monitoring systems store data for easy post hoc analysis and present the original EEG signal together with the aEEG trend. This improves quality control and interpretability.

- Other EEG trends can also be created in the new EEG monitors. They can be used as complementary trends to the aEEG and the EEG.

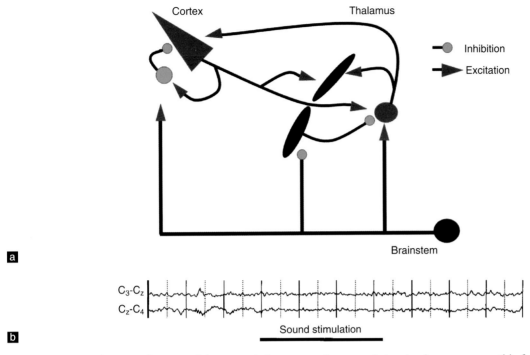

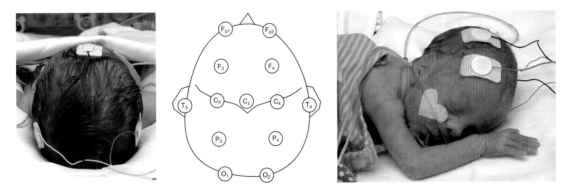

Figure 1.1 (a) Schematic diagram of the main thalamocortical neuronal circuits that are responsible for EEG rhythms. For further details, see text and reference 1.

(b) EEG recording from an awake full-term infant before, during, and after auditory stimulation. Note the reduction of low-frequency EEG components at arousal, during stimulation.

Figure 1.2 The biparietal recording electrodes P3 and P4 have traditionally been the recommended positions for single-channel aEEG. The electrode positions are described according to the international 10–20 system.[18,19] In the 10–20 system, landmarks over the skull are used to determine the placement of electrodes and distances, which are subdivided into 10 or 20% intervals. The vertex is defined as the intersection of the line joining the top of the nose (nasion) to the external occipital protuberance (inion), and the line joining the external auditory meati. In adults P3 and P4 are approximately 5 cm posterior to the vertex and about 8 cm apart. In a full-term neonatal infant the approximate corresponding figures are 3 and 6 cm, respectively. The neutral electrode is positioned anterior in the midline. For two-channel bilateral recording, channels F3–P3 and F4–P4 are recommended. The two photographs above show slightly modified electrode positions, on the left side closest to P3–P4 and on the right side F4–P4.

Priors and Maynard's suggestion for selecting a biparietal derivation for single-channel aEEG monitoring is that the underlying cerebral cortex is in the boundary zone of blood perfusion from the posterior, middle, and cerebral arteries and thus sensitive to ischemia caused by a systemic fall in blood pressure.[9] Whether this is true for newborn infants is not known, although the location is good since it is less affected by scalp muscle activity and eye movement artifacts than temporal or frontal leads.

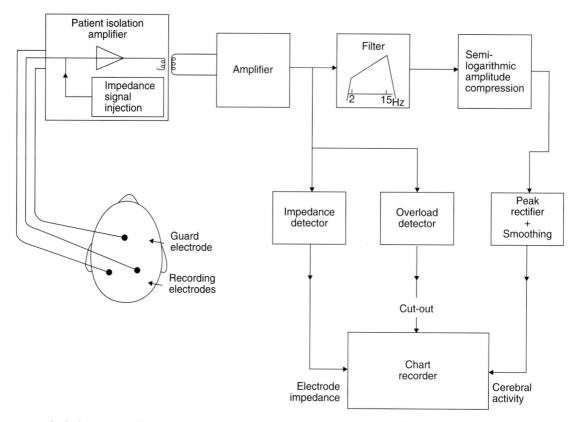

Figure 1.3 Block diagram to show signal pathways in the original CFM (Type 4640). For details, see text. Adapted from reference 9 with permission.

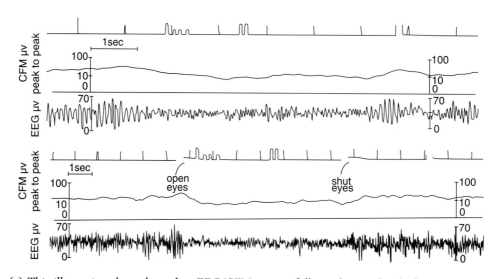

Figure 1.4 (a) This illustration shows how the aEEG/CFM output follows the amplitude fluctuations of the EEG in an awake adult subject. The CFM output has been plotted at the same speed as the EEG instead of at the usual 6 or 30 cm/h. Adapted from reference 9 with permission.

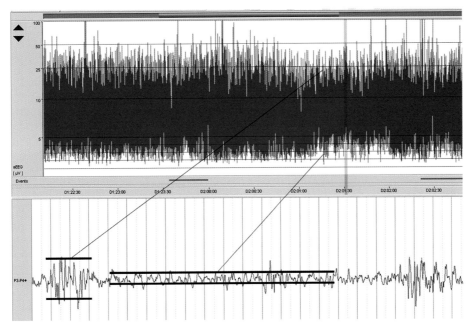

b

(b) Four hours of aEEG and 23 s of the corresponding original EEG in a discontinuous neonatal EEG. The peak-to-peak amplitude of the EEG bursts defines the upper border of the aEEG trace, and the peak-to-peak amplitude of the interburst EEG (duration about 15 s) defines the lower border of the trace. Reproduced from reference 10 with permission.

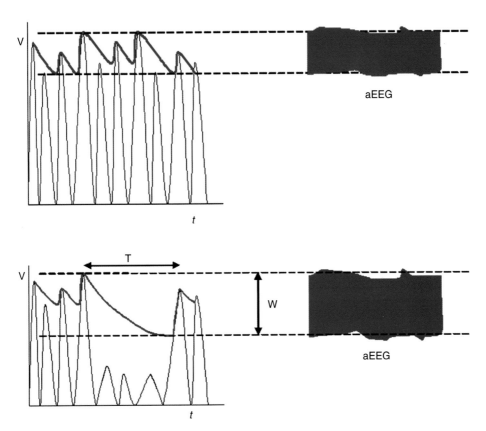

c

Figure 1.4 *opposite and above* (c) Schematic illustration of the effect of the duration of the interburst interval of a discontinuous EEG on the lower border of the aEEG trace. As a result of the time constant of the aEEG display, the lower border of the aEEG trace is determined by both the amplitude and spacing of peaks in the EEG (upper trace). In the presence of repeated discontinuities (IBI = 1–5 s) the position of the lower border is greatly affected by the interburst interval, T (lower trace). Courtesy of Graham McBain, BrainZ Instruments Ltd, Auckland, New Zealand.

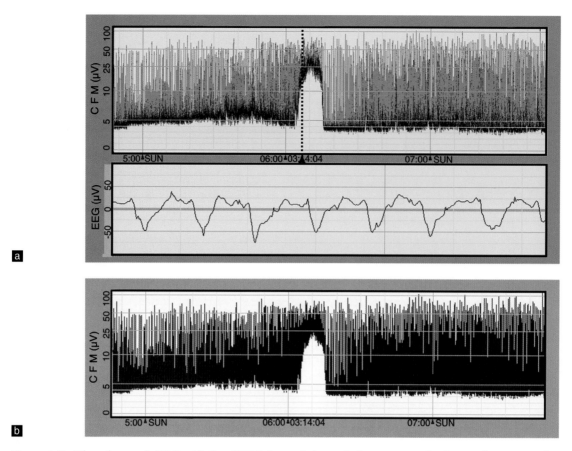

Figure 1.5 Three hours of aEEG with 6 s of EEG from a baby with discontinuous background activity and one seizure with duration around 10 min. Modulation of the gray scale (upper aEEG panel) helps to better define the lower edge of the trace, and the type of background pattern. Also note the 'cap' during the ictal discharge.

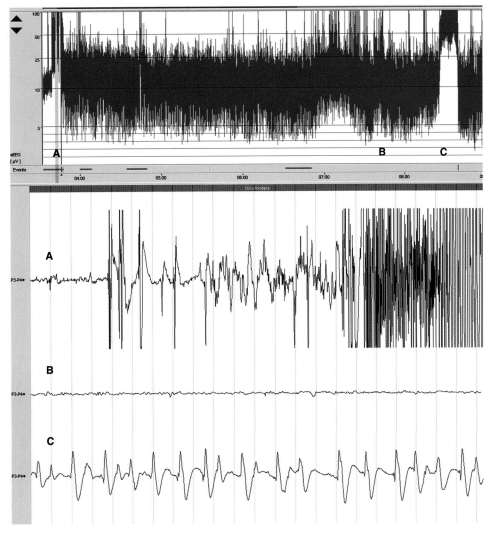

Figure 1.6 This figure shows 5.5 h of mainly continuous aEEG with corresponding 20-s original EEG tracings below. The increased activity in the aEEG at A was caused by a bad electrode, while the similarly increased activity at C was caused by a seizure, as shown by the abrupt onset of a rhythmic ictal EEG pattern that causes a sudden upward shift of the lower and upper border of the aEEG trace. Checking the concomitant EEG makes it possible to safely discriminate this episode of rhythmic epileptic discharges from an artifact caused by movement or a bad electrode (A). The low amplitude interburst EEG is shown in B. Reproduced from reference 10 with permission.

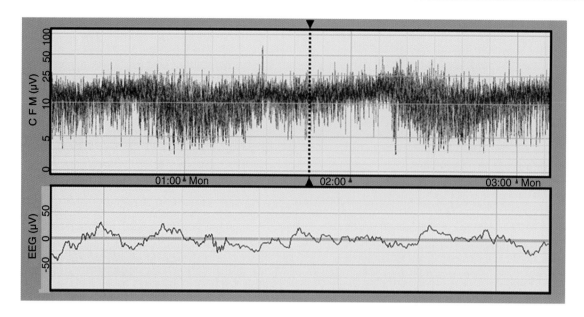

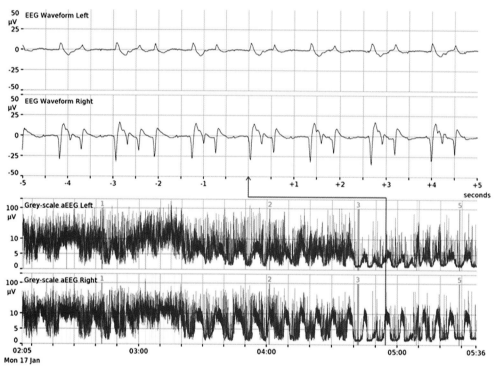

Figure 1.7 This figure demonstrates typical set-ups of the EEG monitors that have been used in the Atlas for most of the examples. These EEG monitors also have other features that can be displayed, as can be seen in the other chapters. Some of the figures that are shown were made from montages from several screen shots.

(a) A recording made by the Olympic Medical CFM 6000 from an asphyxiated term infant after recovery, showing continuous background with sleep–wake cycling. The aEEG trace displays 3 h of recording, and the EEG below shows 6 s. The amplitude scales are shown on the left. The thin narrow vertical lines through the aEEG denote 10-min intervals. The date and time of the recording are shown between the traces. The aEEG at time 01:45 (black stippled vertical line through the aEEG) corresponds to the EEG that is displayed below. In this trace no clinical events were noted.

(b) A recording from a preterm infant with intraventricular hemorrhage and status epilepticus, recorded with the BrainZ BRM2. The two upper panels show 10 s of EEG from the left and right side, respectively. Below are the corresponding aEEGs, displayed with a 3.5 h trend. The red vertical line with arrow shows the part of the aEEG from where the displayed EEG is taken. The green numbered vertical lines mark events.

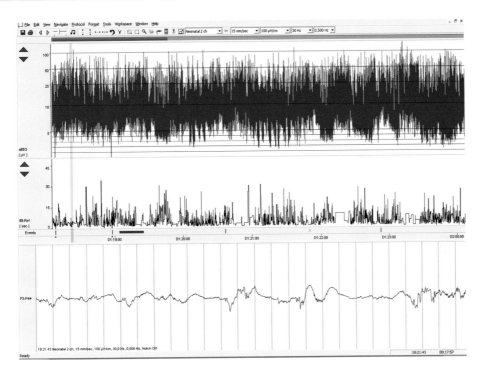

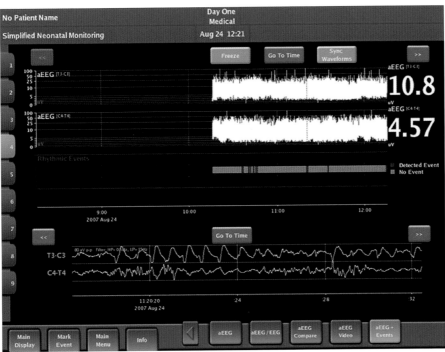

Figure 1.7 *continued* (c) A recording from a stable preterm infant (GA 27w) showing some cyclicity indicative of sleep–wake cycling made with VIASYS NicoletOne. The two upper traces are EEG trends (aEEG and IBI), here with a duration of 6 h (other examples can be 4 h or shorter). The time is shown below the trends as D1:19:00, or day 1 at 19.00 hours. The purple markers above the time scale denote events. Below is 25 s of EEG taken at time 18:21:43 corresponding to the blue vertical line through the trends. The displayed EEG settings are shown right above the aEEG and also in the lower left corner of the EEG.

(d) A full-term infant with slightly discontinuous background and brief seizures displayed on the NEO monitor from Day One Medical. The top of the screen shows two channels of aEEG from a 2-h recording, with the timescale duration set to 4 h. The numbers to the right of the aEEG traces specify the aEEG values at the time corresponding to the dotted red line. Rhythmic events are marked in red on the gray bar under the aEEG trends. The bottom of the screen shows 16 s of EEG corresponding to the dotted red line through the aEEG trends. Courtesy of Damon Lees, Moberg Research, Inc, Ambler, PA, USA.

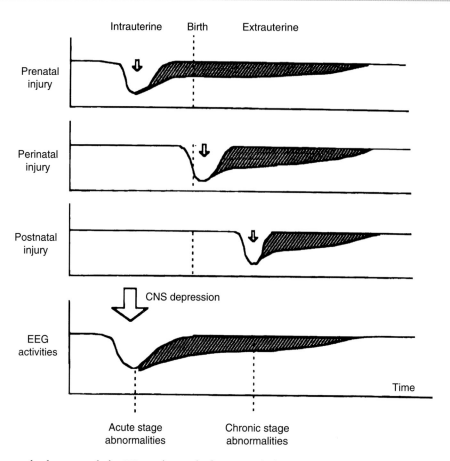

Figure 1.8 Conceptual scheme made by Watanabe et al of acute and chronic consequences on the EEG depending on the timing of perinatal injury in relation to birth. Acute stage abnormalities include depression of electrocortical background activity and increased discontinuity over hours and a few days. Seizures may appear during the early recovery phase. Chronic stage abnormalities include delayed maturation, disorganized background patterns, and the presence of positive rolandic sharp waves (PRSWs), and are seen over weeks and months. The aEEG monitoring is mainly sensitive for acute stage abnormalities. Reproduced from reference 15 with permission.

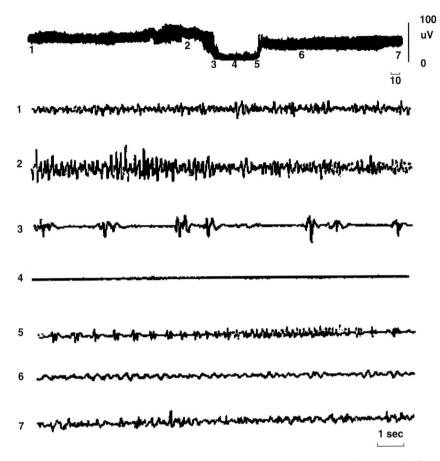

Figure 1.9 Comparison of continuous CFM record and samples of EEG recorded from a rat before, during, and after a period of severe hypoglycemia induced by insulin intraperitoneally. The blood glucose level was restored by iv glucose. For further details see text. Data from reference 16 with permission.

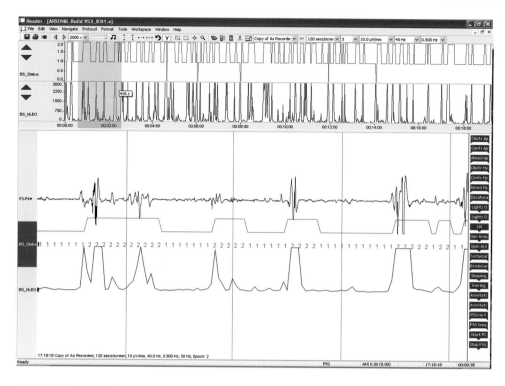

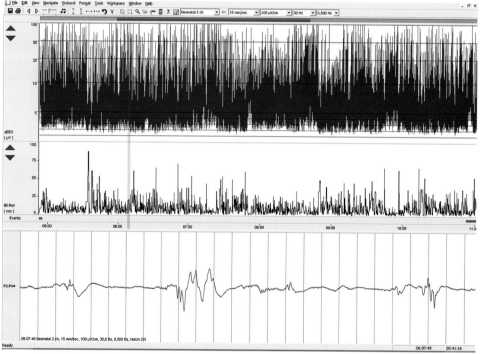

Figure 1.10 (a) Illustration of online categorization of discontinuous EEG into three different states of continuity. From above, the figure shows the following trends during a 20-min period: 'BS_Status' classified as burst (2), suppression (1), or either artifact or continuous (3, not shown). The second panel shows the output from a non-linear energy operator (BS_NLEO). A burst is defined as NLEO > 300 for more than 1 s. Suppression is defined as NLEO < 40 for more than 2 s. If the BS ratio is less than 25%, the signal is considered to be continuous and reports '0' values for BS ratio, IBI, and burst rate. The three lower traces display 120 s of the stippled trends, the upper is the original EEG, 'P3–P4', below is the 'BS_Status' with numbers, and the 'BS_NLEO'. Courtesy of Heidar Einarsson, Viasys Healthcare, Inc, Conshohocken, PA, USA.

(b) Six-hour aEEG and IBI trends from a stable, extremely preterm infant (GA 24 + 4 weeks) recorded a few hours after birth. Below is a representative sample of 25 s of EEG taken at time 06:07 (blue vertical line through trends). The IBI trend enhances identification of fluctuations in the electrocortical background which are not easily detected in the aEEG trace alone.

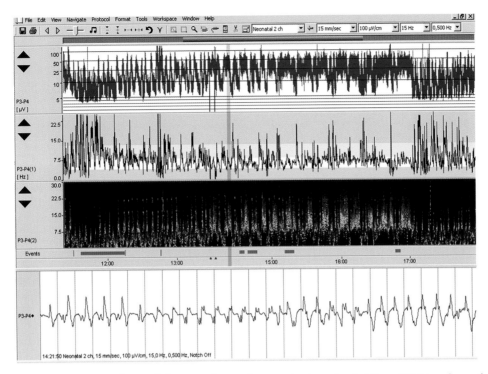

Figure 1.11 This is a 6-h recording from a full-term infant with severe birth asphyxia. Three EEG trends are shown above the 25 s of EEG corresponding to the gray vertical line through the EEG trends, from top and down: aEEG–95% SEF–spectrogram. The subclinical status epilepticus that is present during the whole recording is visible in all trends, but is most evident in the aEEG. The amplitude depression during the last hour of recording is due to administration of antiepileptic medication.

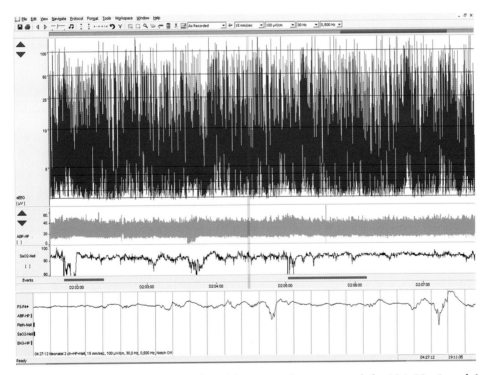

Figure 1.12 A 6-h polygraphic trend monitoring of a stable, extremely premature baby (GA 23+6 weeks) starting during the first 12 h. From above the aEEG, blood pressure and oxygen saturation trends are displayed. Some instability is seen in the oxygen saturation trend, especially in connection with care procedures (green horizontal lines). The 25 s of EEG below shows a discontinuous *tracé dicontinu* pattern from time 04:27 (blue vertical line through the trends). The blood pressure curve, the signal from the oxygen saturation monitor, and the ECG below the EEG have been omitted in the 25-s sequence to increase the visibility of the EEG.

2

The electrocortical background, its normal maturation, classification, and effects of medication

MATURATION

The EEG can be recorded in newborns at all maturational levels, also in the extremely preterm infants. The understanding and correct interpretation of the neonatal EEG is based on knowledge of the normal development of the EEG from early preterm stages to the postterm period, and associated maturational time cues. This also includes variations in EEG patterns related to different stages of the sleep–wake cycle (AS, QS, W). When discussing maturational features of the newborn EEG, several terms have been used to define the maturity of the infant: newborn infants are born at a certain gestational age (GA), their postnatal age (PNA) increases after birth, as does their postmenstrual age (PMA) or postconceptional/conceptional age (PCA/CA). The PMA and PCA/CA are summaries of the gestational age plus the postnatal age in weeks. PCA and CA are terms that are commonly used in the EEG literature.

The development and normal EEG maturation in moderately preterm and term infants have been described in detail.[20-25] Current knowledge about the normal EEG of the extremely low GA infant is more limited since only a few studies have included long-term follow-up.[26]

A model for explaining the EEG ontogeny has recently been proposed, including a superimposition of two developmental trajectories.[5] The first component is the repetitive occurrence of high-amplitude bursts of activity superimposed on low-frequency waves of high amplitude (SATs) (see Figure 2.1). SATs are generated already at a CA of 24 weeks; they become roughly coincident between hemispheres at around 30 weeks' gestation but attain a more consistent

temporal synchrony only later, from about 35 weeks' GA. The amplitude of SATs gradually decreases with maturation, and they are not normally present at term. The duration of SATs increases with maturation. The second component is a gradual development of continuous oscillatory EEG activity that is dependent on the development of functional thalamocortical and intracortical connections during the third trimester until about 40–50 weeks of CA. This component is virtually absent in the very premature infant.

As a result of these developmental processes the normal EEG background of the very preterm infant is discontinuous (in the EEG literature this pattern is often called *tracé discontinu*) (Figures 2.2 and 2.3). With increasing maturation the periods with low voltage activity, called IBIs, become shorter. In parallel, the duration of the bursts increases with a decrease in burst amplitude so that the overall background activity becomes continuous in the awake state (Figure 2.4).[27] This development occurs also in extremely preterm infants, as shown in Figure 2.5.[28] Table 2.1 summarizes data on average and maximum IBIs at different postmenstrual ages obtained from several studies.[26-31] For comparison, the automated IBI that was averaged from artifact-free periods during several hours over the first 72 hours of life in eight infants of 24 to 28 weeks' GA who were healthy at 2 years of age was 8.7 s.[32] Reference values for the number of bursts/hour in very preterm infants were evaluated in aEEGs from a cohort of 75 preterm infants with of 23 to 29 weeks' GA.[33] The median number of bursts/hour during the first week of life was: 20.4 (GA 24–25 weeks), 14.9 (GA 26–27 weeks), and 4.4 (GA 28–29 weeks).

A few studies indicate that the electrocortical background undergoes more subtle maturational

Table 2.1 Mean and maximum IBIs in healthy preterm and near-term infants as recorded with intermittent EEG (data modified from references 26–31)

Postconceptional age (weeks)	Mean IBI (s)	Maximum IBI (s)
21–22	26	
23–24	18	
25–27	12	35–45
28–30	10–12	30–35
31–33	8–10	20
34–36	6–8	10
37–40		6

changes as well during the first days of life in very preterm infants, which can be evaluated by estimating continuity and power spectral measures.[34–36]

With the aEEG technique it is possible to record cerebral activity for prolonged periods of time from full-term and preterm infants. The main features that can be extracted from the aEEG include:

- The type of background activity in terms of discontinuous/continuous activity;

- An estimate of IBIs or burst rate;

- Cyclic variation in the background activity corresponding to sleep–wake cycling; and

- The presence of EEG seizure patterns.

However, complete information about hemispheric side asymmetries and synchrony, frequency content of EEG bursts, and the occurrence of specific EEG features of clinical and prognostic significance such as delta brushes, positive rolandic sharp waves, temporal sharp waves, or other interictal sharp transients cannot be obtained with the reduced number of electrodes used for EEG monitoring, and a standard EEG is recommended when such information is warranted.

Sleep–wake cycling comprises cyclic alterations in behavioral states that can be evaluated based on observations of eye movements, respiration, muscle tone, and movements. Although the exact correlations with sleep stages later in life are not fully delineated, these state changes are also associated with changes in the EEG patterns that are usually clearly discernible in the aEEG trace. Cyclic variations in the aEEG background, presumably reflecting cyclic alterations between periods of QS and periods of AS/W can be seen in well infants from around 25–26 weeks'

PCA[37,38] (Figure 2.6). From around 30–31 gestational weeks QS periods are readily distinguished in the aEEG trace as periods of 20–30 minutes' duration with increased bandwidth (Figure 2.7);[38] at full term these periods represent the *tracé alternant* EEG pattern (Figure 2.8).

CLASSIFICATION

A number of publications, two of them published in 1984, have described the normal development of aEEG patterns in full-term and preterm infants.[11,13,33,39,40] Thornberg and Thiringer presented a study on normal aEEG development in preterm and full-term infants who had an uneventful neonatal period and were neurologically normal at follow-up.[38] Normative data for minimum and maximum amplitudes during wakefulness and sleep were included in their evaluation. The aEEG feature most clearly related to maturation in healthy infants was the lower edge (amplitude) of the quiet sleep trace.[11,38] As seen in Figure 2.9, the amplitude of the minimum EEG activity, mainly representing the level of activity between high amplitude bursts, gradually increases with maturation, reflecting the continuous development of oscillatory EEG generators (see above).

Burdjalov et al studied 30 infants (GA 24–39 weeks) serially on 146 occasions, twice during the first 3 days of life and then weekly or biweekly.[41] A scoring system evaluating continuity, cyclic (sleep–wake cycling) changes, and amplitude of lower border and bandwidth was applied to the recordings (Figure 2.10). The range of the summarized score points was 0–13. The total score showed a very good correlation with GA and PCA; the highest total score was attained at 35–36 weeks' PCA. Abnormal patterns, e.g. burst-suppression or seizures, were not included in the scoring system.

Al Naqeeb et al created a classification including three categories for normal and abnormal aEEGs in full-term infants.[42] The classification is based on aEEG amplitudes, and 14 healthy controls defined the normal pattern. In the healthy infants the median upper margin of the widest band of aEEG activity was 37.5 μV (range 30–48 μV), and the median lower margin was 8 μV (range 6.5–11 μV). The aEEG background activity was classified as normal amplitude when the upper margin of the aEEG activity was >10 μV and the lower margin was >5 μV; moderately abnormal when the upper margin of aEEG was >10 μV and the lower margin was <5 μV; and suppressed when the upper margin of the aEEG was <10 μV and the lower margin was <5 μV. Seizure activity was defined, but not sleep–wake cycling. This classification was recently used in a randomized multicenter study evaluating the effect of postasphyxia head cooling.[43]

Several models for classification of aEEG patterns have been suggested. It is obvious that some classifications are relevant only for a certain group of NICU patients, e.g. asphyxiated full-term or normal preterm infants. We therefore proposed a classification of aEEG background patterns, based on EEG terminology, including categorization of sleep–wake cycling, which could be used in all newborn infants (see Tables 2.2 and 2.3, and Figure 2.11).[44] In this proposal we have used and modified some of the classifications described above. The classification does not include evaluation of background patterns and amplitudes in relation to normative data for different GAs. Similar to basic EEG interpretation, we suggest that pattern recognition also forms the basis for interpretation of the aEEG trace (Figure 2.12).

The amplitude of the electrocortical activity is, of course, extremely important, but this measure must be handled with caution since it can be affected by extracerebral artifacts and by interelectrode distance,

Table 2.2 Classification of aEEG background patterns

The background pattern describes the dominating type of electrocortical activity in the aEEG trace:

- Continuous (C): continuous activity with lower (minimum) amplitude around (5)–7–10 μV, and maximum amplitudes 10–25(–50) μV. This pattern is often called a continuous normal voltage (CNV) pattern in full-term infants.

- Discontinuous (DC): discontinuous activity with minimum amplitude variable, but mainly below 5 μV, and maximum amplitudes over 10 μV.

- Continuous low voltage (CLV): continuous activity of very low amplitude (around or below 5 μV).

- Burst-suppression (BS): discontinuous activity with minimum amplitude without variability at 0–1 (2) μV, and bursts with amplitude >25 μV.

  - BS+ denotes a BS background with dense bursts ≥ 100 bursts/h;

  - BS– defines a BS background with sparse bursts, < 100 bursts/h.

- Inactive, flat (FT): Mainly inactive background (electrocerebral inactivity) below 5 μV.

Table 2.3 Classification of sleep–wake cycling

Sleep–wake cycling (SWC) in the aEEG is characterized by smooth cyclic variations, mainly of the minimum amplitude (i.e. lower border). Periods with broader bandwidth represent more discontinuous activity during quiet sleep (*tracé alternant* in full-term infants), and the narrower parts of the trace correspond to more continuous background during wakefulness or active sleep.

- No SWC: no sinusoidal variations of the aEEG background.

- Imminent/immature SWC: some, but not fully developed, cyclic variation of the lower border amplitude, but not developed as compared to normative maturational age-matched data.

- Developed SWC: clearly identifiable sinusoidal changes between discontinuous and more continuous background in the aEEG with cycle duration ≥ 20 min.

as further discussed in Chapters 1 and 3. Close inspection of the original EEG trace, which accompanies the aEEG trace in modern equipment, is highly recommended in order to exclude some sources for artifacts. Nevertheless, normative values for minimum and maximum amplitudes of the aEEG at different GAs have been published.[11,36,39,40,42] They can be very helpful in assisting the evaluation of aEEG recordings in relation to what can be expected for a certain maturational age. As mentioned above, the minimum amplitude during QS periods is particularly valuable to assess since it increases with GA up to term. Furthermore, short-term variability of the minimum amplitude is a sign separating a discontinuous EEG from a burst suppression (BS) pattern. As demonstrated in Figure 1.4c (Chapter 1), at short IBIs the level of the lower border of the aEEG trace is influenced by both the amplitude of the bursts as well as the amplitude of EEG activity between the bursts.

aEEG AND MEDICATIONS

A common clinical dilemma is that a baby treated with antiepileptic or sedative medications also needs to have the EEG recorded. Sedative and antiepileptic medications often affect and depress the electrocortical background activity, thereby obscuring the 'true' status of the brain. If the EEG background is considered normal there is usually no problem with the interpretation. However, often the EEG background is more discontinuous and depressed than what could be expected for the conceptional age, and in these cases the clinician and the neurophysiologist must distinguish what could be a real sign of abnormal brain function from, e.g., previous hypoxia–ischemia, or an effect from previously given medications. Several studies have evaluated drug effects on the neonatal EEG. However, it is not possible and ethically justified to administer medications to healthy newborns just to evaluate effects on the EEG, and therefore there are methodologic problems with these studies since the medications were usually given to sick infants on clinical indications.

In general, most sedative and antiepileptic drugs depress electrocortical background activity, including sleep–wake cycling. The degree of background depression is associated with the type of medication, the dose, and the time the drug was given in relation to the EEG.[45–49] The EEG response to some medications also seems to be associated with illness severity. Healthier babies seem to respond less than severely ill neonates and infants with severe hypoxic–ischemic brain injury, although this has not been formally evaluated in any study. Most of the current knowledge about drug effects on the EEG background is derived from studies using continuous EEG monitoring (see below).

The effects on the EEG from small bolus doses and continuous infusion of opioids such as morphine and fentanyl seem to be only minor in term infants and moderately preterm infants. Phenobarbital loading doses and phenobarbital treatment with concentrations within therapeutic levels also appear to affect the EEG background only moderately.[12] Phenobarbital does not seem to obscure evaluation of the EEG background pattern in term infants after moderate birth asphyxia. Continuous EEG background may become slightly–moderately discontinuous, while the EEG background in infants with more severe birth asphyxia and discontinuous EEG may react more, e.g. change into BS or low voltage. Furthermore, the therapeutic concentration of phenobarbital does not appear to affect the predictive sensitivity of the aEEG background in preterm infants with grade 3–4 IVHs.[50] When using long-term EEG monitoring it is clear that there is variability in the EEG background; effects from boluses of medications such as phenobarbital, phenytoin, diazepam, midazolam, and morphine mainly affect the EEG background 1–2 h after medications have been administered.

Administration of the antiepileptic medication lidocaine quite often leads to BS both in term and in preterm infants. However, lidocaine is usually given when other medications such as phenobarbital and midazolam/diazepam failed to control seizures, and the effect on the EEG background may be influenced by the added effects of the medications. Nevertheless, we have seen rather abrupt shifts from BS to slightly discontinuous background when lidocaine was discontinued after it had been tailored off for certain hours.

Endotracheal administration of surfactant for respiratory distress syndrome sometimes results in a short, but very profound, depression of electrocortical activity which may become transiently inactive for about 10 minutes.[51] The mechanism for this reaction is not known. Some studies indicate that the electrocortical background may also become affected by carbon dioxide levels and by cardiac output, although the mechanisms by which these conditions affect the electrocortical activity are more on a hemodynamic level, and are more closely related to hypoxic–ischemic brain injury.[52–55]

Practical recommendations for aEEG/EEG recording and interpretation in relation to medication are summarized in Table 2.4.

Table 2.4 Recommendations for interpretation of aEEG/EEG in infants receiving sedatives, opioid analgesics or antiepileptic medications

- Sedatives, opioids, and antiepileptic medications may all depress the electrocortical activity and render it more discontinuous than it was, i.e. a continuous background may become slightly discontinuous, and an already discontinuous background may change into BS, and a BS background may develop a more sparse burst pattern, or become flat.

- Evaluation of the aEEG/EEG background activity may become uncertain for 1–2 h following administration of sedatives and opioid analgesics. On the other hand, the long-term aEEG trend monitoring enhances identification of such effects on the electrocortical activity.

- Moderate doses of sedatives and analgesics usually do not result in severe or long-lasting depression of the aEEG/EEG background, unless the baby is very immature or very ill with already compromised brain function.

SUMMARY

- The electrocortical background activity develops from a discontinuous EEG in the very preterm infant to a predominantly continuous EEG in the term infant. This development is reflected in the aEEG trend patterns.

- Cycling between different activity states (sleep–wake cycle) is reflected in the aEEG, and can be seen in stable infants from around 25 weeks' PCA.

- A suggested model for classification of the aEEG background pattern in well and sick neonates is presented.

- The user of aEEG must be aware of the fact that a number of antiepileptic, sedative, and anesthetic agents may influence the aEEG background patterns.

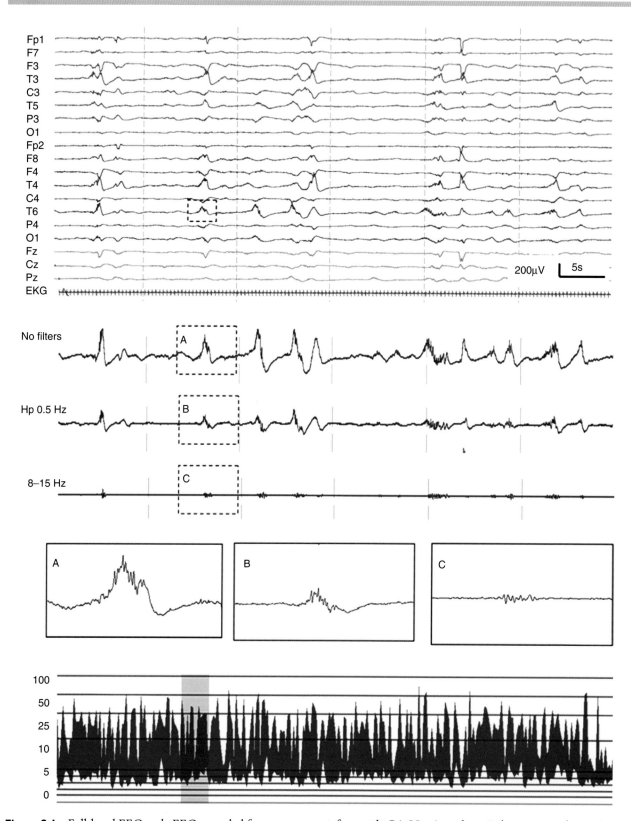

Figure 2.1 Full-band EEG and aEEG recorded from a preterm infant with GA 32 + 4 weeks at 2 days postnatal age. Apgar scores were 3, 5, and 7. The infant had a small intraventricular hemorrhage (IVH II). The upper graph shows full 10–20 electrode array in a Laplacian montage in order to illustrate the spatial organization of the EEG. The EEG trace from electrode T6 (dashed rectangle) is displayed below the full-band EEG and shown with different filters: ('No filters'), conventional EEG filters ('Hp 0.5 Hz'), and with filters similar to aEEG ('8–15 Hz'). The gray bar in the aEEG trace below represents the displayed EEG epoch above. Figure provided by courtesy of Sampsa Vanhatalo.

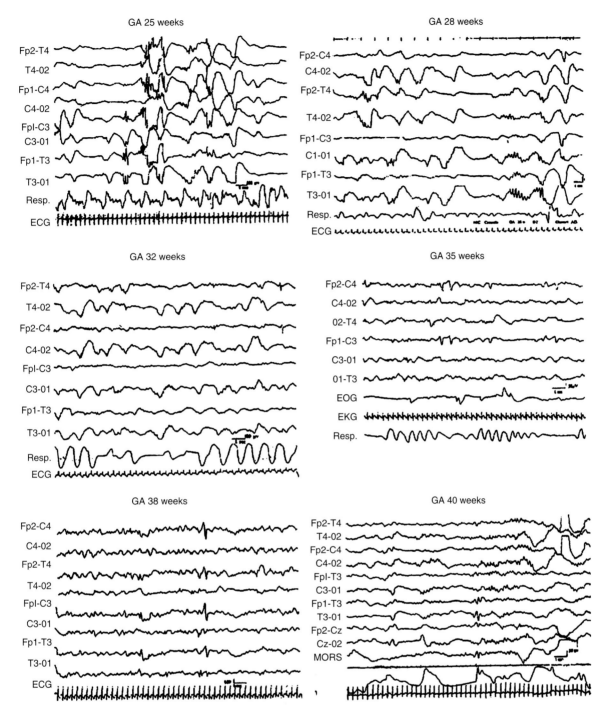

Figure 2.2 The figure shows development of continuous EEG activity, representing active sleep (AS) and/or periods of wakefulness (W), at different GAs. At 25 weeks' GA the EEG is predominantly discontinuous with only brief (<60 s) periods of continuous activity. From 28 weeks' GA the periods of continuous activity become longer and more frequent. From 32 weeks' gestation and onwards AS and W stages show a continuous EEG pattern. From reference 24 with permission.

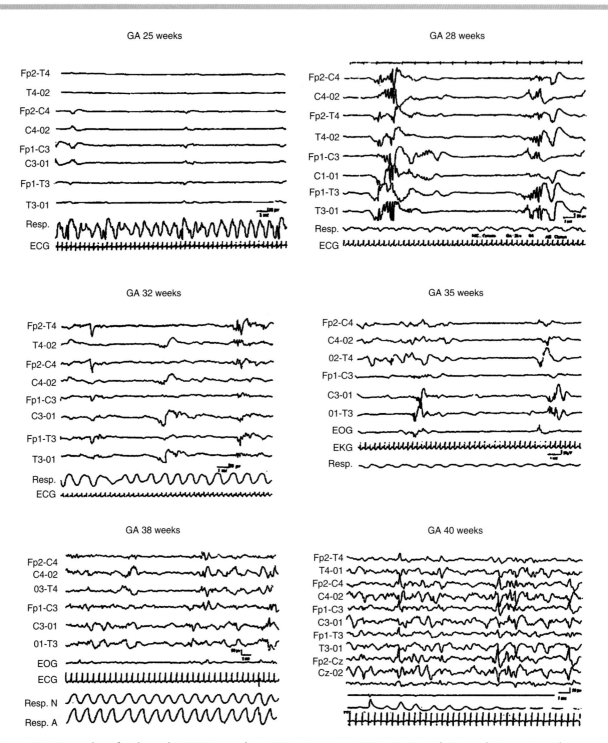

Figure 2.3 Examples of polygraphic EEG records in QS at increasing GA. At 25 and 28 weeks' gestation the trace is very discontinuous. At 32 and 35 weeks' GA, a *tracé discontinu* pattern is seen with decreasing IBIs gradually changing into a *tracé alternant* pattern at term. From reference 24 with permission.

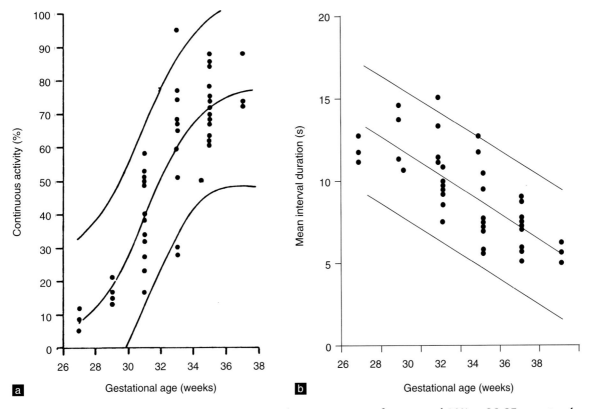

Figure 2.4   (a) Development of continuous EEG activity during maturation from around 10% at 26–27 gestational weeks to 70–80% at term.

(b) Development of IBI duration with GA. Measurements were made from the most discontinuous quiet-sleep parts in 45 recordings from infants of 26–37 weeks' GA using a four-channel Oxford Medilog recorder. From reference 27 with permission.

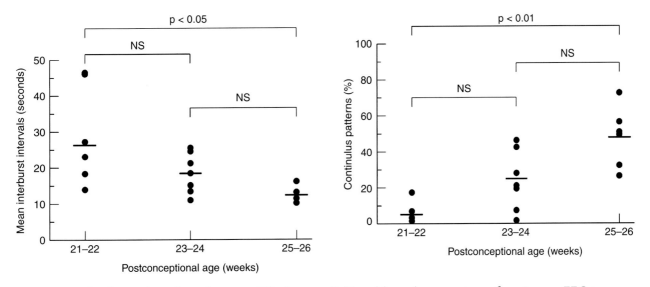

Figure 2.5   This figure shows how the mean IBIs decrease (left) and how the percentage of continuous EEG increases (right) in three groups of extremely immature infants of GA between 21 and 26 weeks. NS, non-significant. From reference 28 with permission.

aEEG in very preterm infants

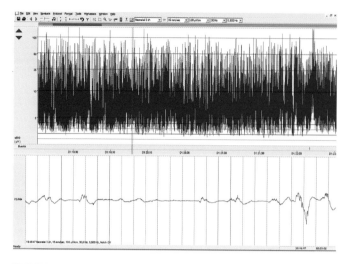

a GA: 22+6 weeks

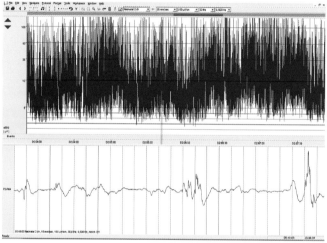

b GA: 23+4 weeks

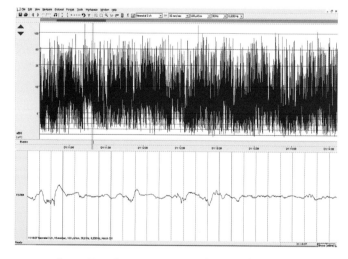

c GA: 23+6 weeks

Figure 2.6 aEEG in very preterm infants. Four-hour aEEG recordings with 25 s of representative EEG activity from the first 2 days of life in eight infants with GAs: (a) 22+6 weeks; (b) 23+4 weeks; (c) 23+6 weeks; (d) 24+2 weeks; (e) 25+3 weeks; (f) 26+3 weeks; (g) 27+3 weeks; (h) 28+4 weeks; and (i) 30+1 weeks. None of the infants had IVH (although the infant in (a) later developed an IVH grade 3). The aEEG pattern is mainly discontinuous in traces (a)–(f), but traces (g) and (h) contain significant amounts of continuous activity. No seizures were detected. A cyclical pattern suggestive of crude sleep–wake cycling can be seen in traces (b), (e), (f), (g), (h) and (i).

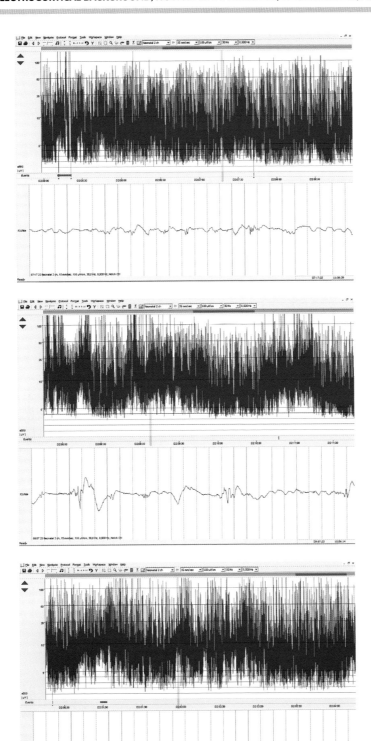

d GA: 24+2 weeks

e GA: 25+3 weeks

f GA: 26+3 weeks

Figure 2.6 *opposite and above*

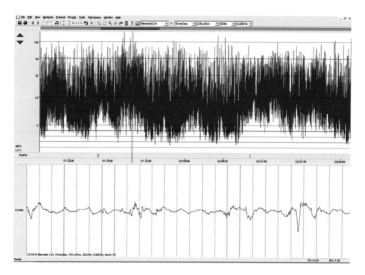

g GA: 27+3 weeks

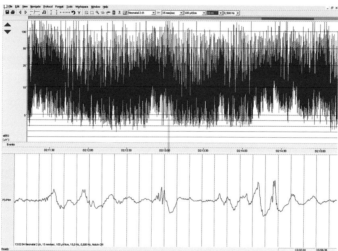

h GA: 28+4 weeks

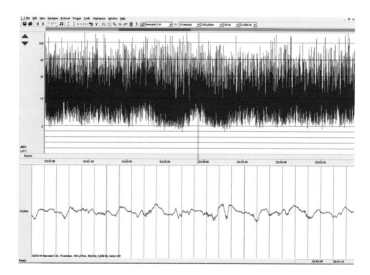

i GA: 30+1 weeks

Figure 2.6 *continued*

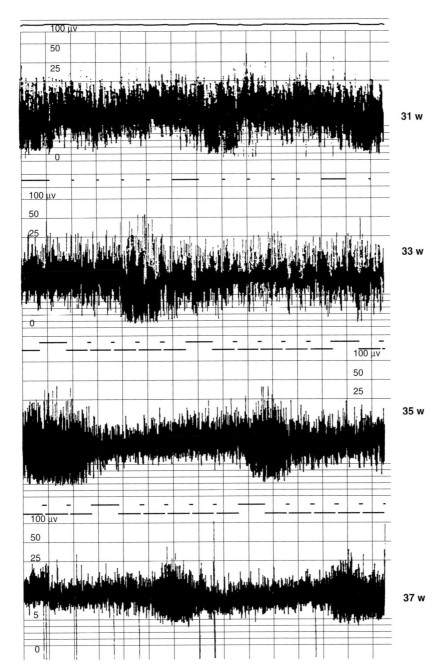

Figure 2.7 Consecutive recordings of aEEG by the CFM from 31 to 37 weeks' postconceptional age (PCA) in an infant born at 30 weeks' gestation. Periods of QS, with more discontinuous EEG activity, can be seen in the aEEG record as periods with 'broad bands', i.e. large minimum–maximum amplitude differences. This can be compared to the more narrow periods representing continuous EEG during active sleep or wakefulness (these two states cannot be distinguished by the aEEG only). Note the transient increase in minimum amplitudes during QS, initially close to zero at 31 and 33 weeks (*tracé discontinu*), later to levels around 5 µV at 37 weeks (*tracé alternant*). From reference 39 with permission.

aEEG and EEG during wakefulness and quiet sleep

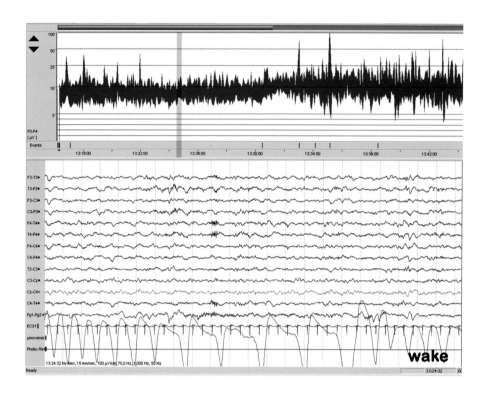

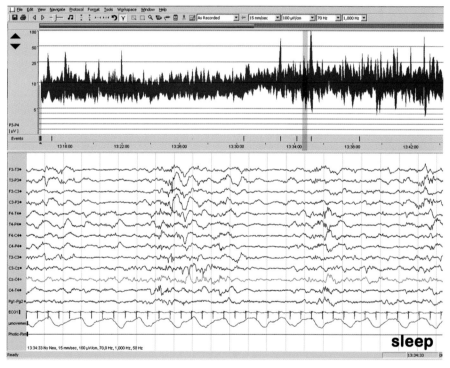

Figure 2.8 aEEG and EEG during wakefulness and quiet sleep. Full EEG recording of a healthy full-term baby, during W (above) and during QS (bottom). The aEEG (duration 27 minutes) was derived from the EEG recording. A *tracé alternant* pattern is recorded during QS, identified in the aEEG as a period with increased amplitude bandwidth. Slow-wave sleep is also present during QS periods in full-term infants, and is usually seen in the aEEG as periods with increased discontinuity and broader bandwidth, similar to the *tracé alternant*.

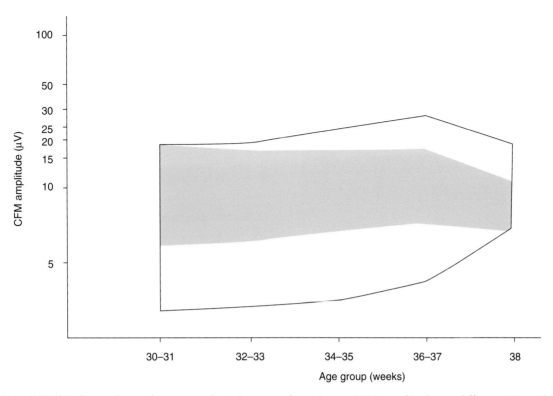

Figure 2.9 (a) This figure shows the expected minimum and maximum CFM amplitudes at different GAs. The white area shows the variation of the broadest bandwidth (corresponding to QS), the stippled area the narrowest bandwidth (corresponding to AS and W). From reference 39 with permission.

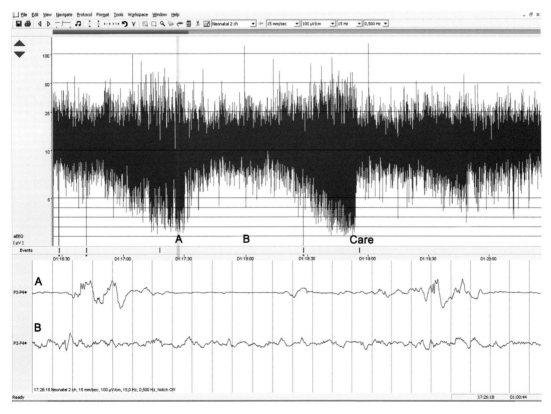

(b) This recording from a moderately preterm infant, born at 35 gestational weeks but with a Dandy-Walker malformation and hydrocephalus, shows a mainly continuous aEEG background with slightly 'clumsy' sleep–wake cycling with very discontinuous QS periods. A care procedure interrupted the second QS period just before time 19:00.

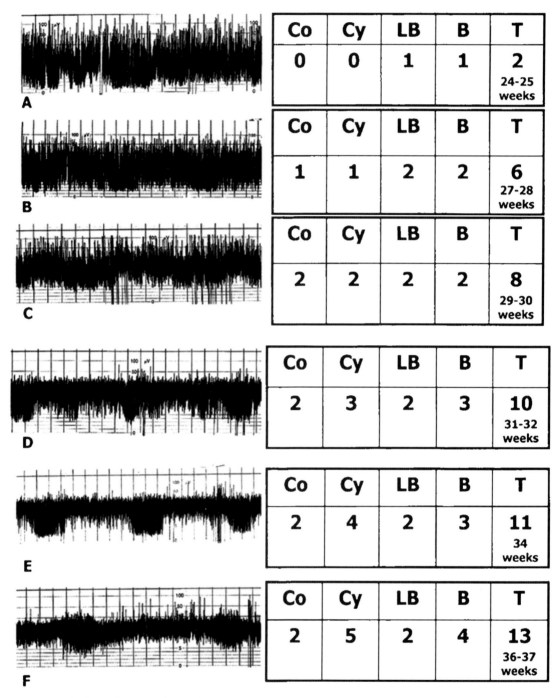

Figure 2.10 (a) The left side of the figure demonstrates how CFM recordings can be scored to assess brain maturation by estimating: Co = continuity, Cy = presence of cycling, LB = lower border amplitude score, B = bandwidth, and T = total summary score of the previous variables. The examples show CFM tracings from normal infants with increasing (from A through F) PCA. From reference 41 with permission.

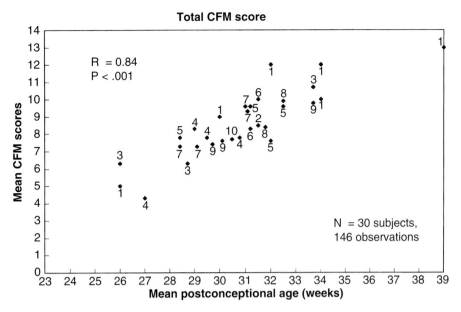

Figure 2.10 (b) Correlation between mean total score and increasing maturation between 24 and 39 weeks' PCA. The total number of studies was 146. There are multiple overlapping points at intersections of mean CFM score and postconceptional age, with the number of studies at each point indicated. From reference 41 with permission.

aEEG background patterns

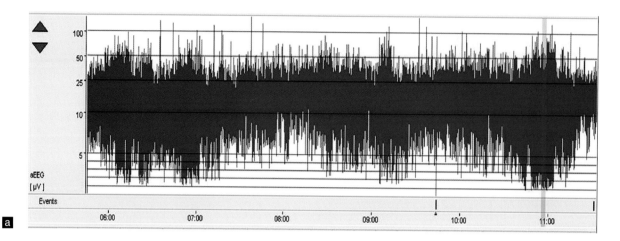

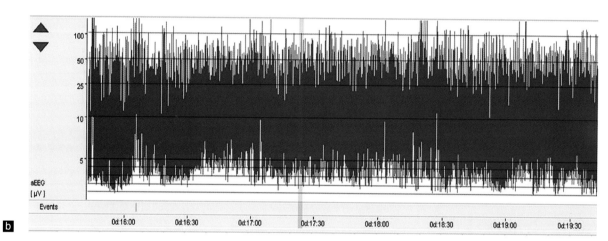

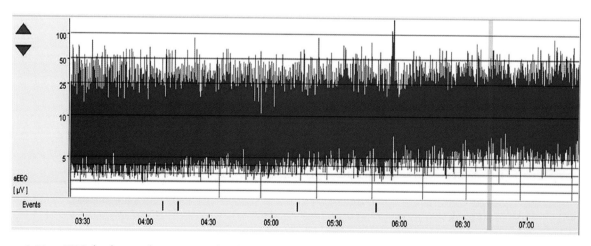

Figure 2.11 aEEG background patterns. Classification of aEEG background patterns (duration of traces 4–6 hours): (a) continuous normal voltage with sleep–wake cycling (C); (b) discontinuous (DC); (c) DC gradually becoming more continuous; (d) burst suppression with high burst density (BS+); (e) burst suppression with low burst density (BS–); (f) continuous extremely low voltage (CLV); (g) inactive, flat (FT). For definitions please see text, Table 2.2 and reference 44.

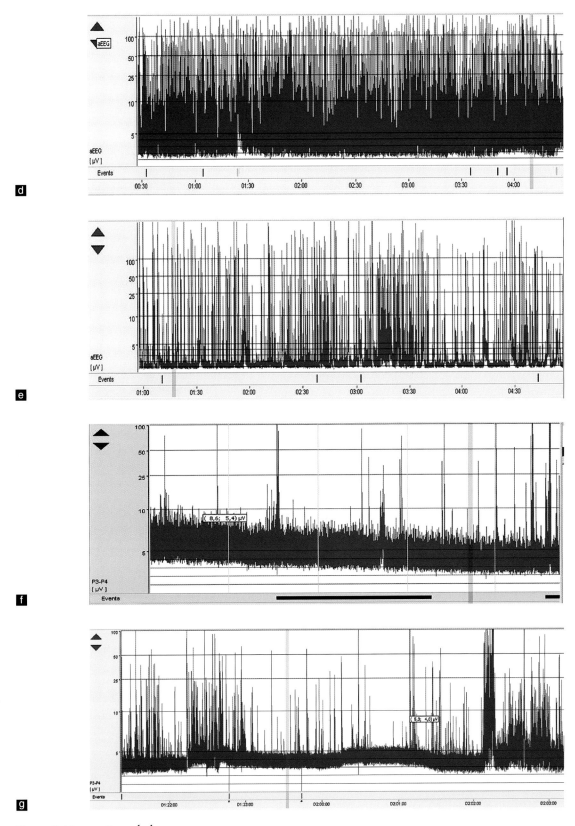

Figure 2.11 *opposite and above*

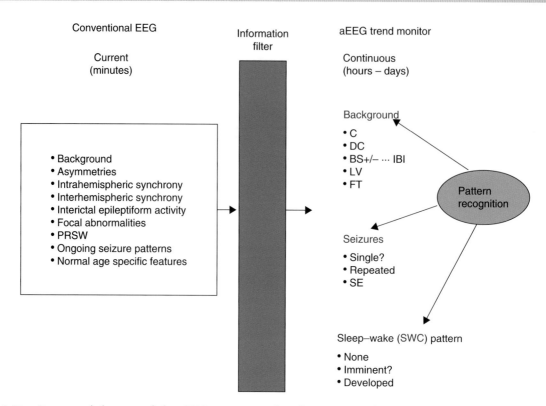

Figure 2.12 Conceptual diagram of the aEEG as compared with conventional EEG. The aEEG helps in continuously extracting three features – background activity (C, continuous; DC, discontinuous; BS+/–, burst suppression with dense or sparse burst activity; IBI, inter burst interval; LV, low voltage; FT, flat), sleep–wake cycling, and ictal patterns (SE, status epilepticus) – that have been proven to be relevant for prognosis and treatment of the preterm and sick term newborn.

Effect of phenobarbitone in two full-term infants

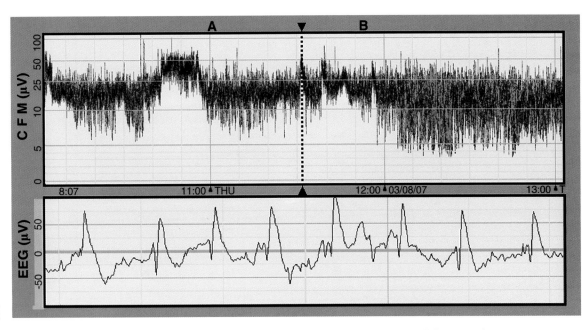

Effect of a loading dose of phenobarbitone (20 mg/kg intravenously) is shown in two full-term infants.

(a) This infant had a right-sided middle cerebral artery infarct (see Figure 6.1 for the full history). Following development of clinical hemiconvulsions a loading dose of phenobarbitone was administered (marker B), which changed the background pattern to a more discontinuous pattern, as reflected by the lower minimum amplitude. The background activity recovered over the following 3 h to a continuous pattern.

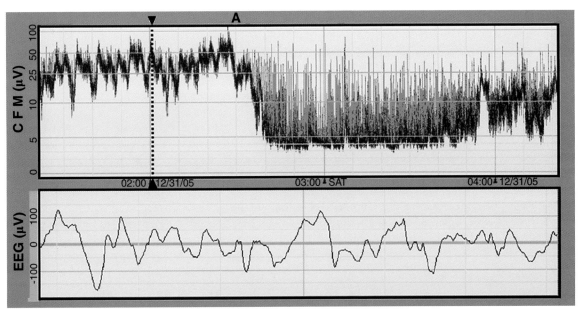

Figure 2.13 (b) In the second infant with severe hypoxic–ischemic encephalopathy (HIE), a 'saw-tooth' pattern, corresponding to status epilepticus, was present at the beginning of the recording. The underlying background pattern is difficult to see, as there is no full recovery in between the seizures. After phenobarbitone (marker A) the electrographic seizure pattern ceased and the background changed to a burst-suppression pattern. Recurrence of ictal discharges is seen at the end of the panel (see Figure 5.8 for full case). There was a drift of the baseline; the minimum level of the aEEG activity should (probably) be lower than 5 μV. The raised baseline could be explained by ECG artifact, which is often seen in patients with very low voltage aEEG activity.

Effect of midazolam in a full-term asphyxiated infant

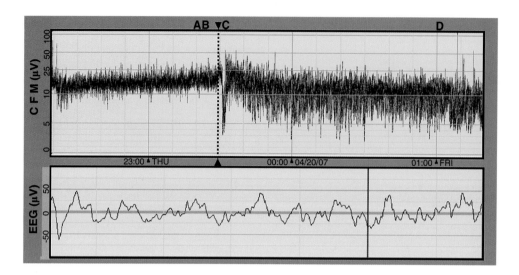

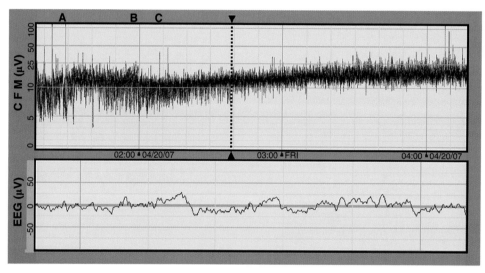

Figure 2.14 This female infant was born at 42 weeks by an emergency Cesarean section following a persistent bradycardia on the cardiotogram (CTG). Apgar scores were 1, 6, and 7 at 1, 5, and 10 minutes, respectively, and the umbilical artery pH was 6.86 with a base excess of −20 mmol/l. She had a clinical seizure in the local hospital and was given a loading dose of phenobarbitone before referral to the regional NICU. She was treated with a loading dose of midazolam (0.5 mg/kg) following a period of suspected subtle seizures (hiccups and lipsmacking), that were not confirmed by the single-channel aEEG or EEG. The loading dose was not calculated correctly and instead of 0.05 mg/kg, 0.5 mg/kg was given iv at C. A very short and acute decrease in aEEG amplitude was noted associated with an apnea, followed by a persistent mild depression of the background pattern, from continuous normal voltage to a mildly discontinuous pattern (a). Two doses of flumazenil, to reverse the effects of the midazolam, were given and, following the second dose, the background pattern normalized, although without any sleep–wake cycling (b).

This example illustrates that even a high dose of midazolam does not always result in a severely depressed background pattern. In the absence of moderate to severe underlying neurologic problems the effect can be mild and transient. The example also shows that the aEEG/EEG or standard EEG should verify the epileptic nature of clinically suspected seizures before administration of antiepileptic medications.

Effect of morphine and diazepam in a preterm infant

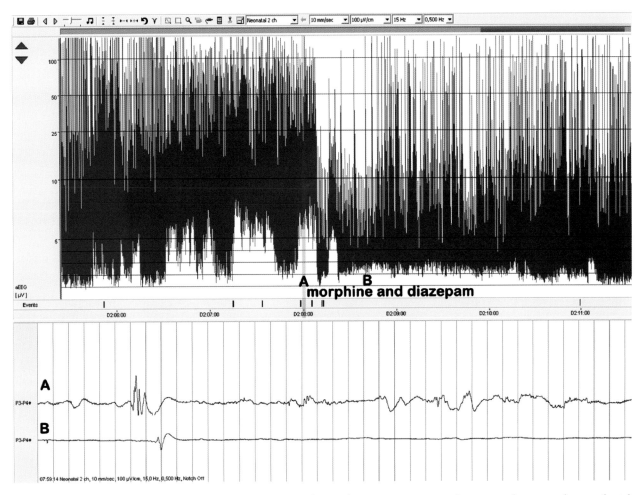

Figure 2.15 This extremely preterm infant (GA 26 weeks) with severe respiratory distress syndrome, and treated with mechanical ventilation, received diazepam and morphine which resulted in a long-lasting suppression (more than 3 h) of the aEEG background. The two EEG traces below (38 s) represent the electrocortical activity before (A) the medications, and after (B).

Effect of lidocaine in a full-term infant with HIE

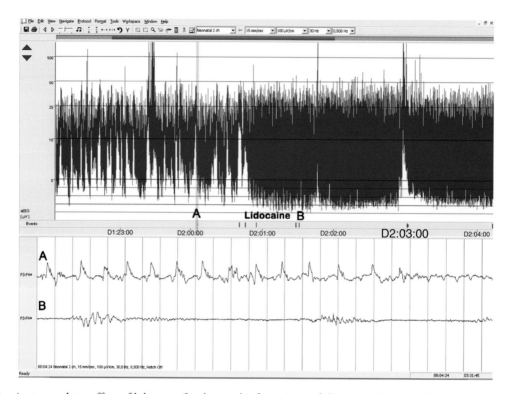

Figure 2.16 Anticonvulsive effect of lidocaine (loading and infusion), in a full-term asphyxiated baby with status epilepticus who was already receiving phenobarbitone and midazolam. The increase in aEEG amplitude at 03:00 is due to care.

Trend measures of continuity

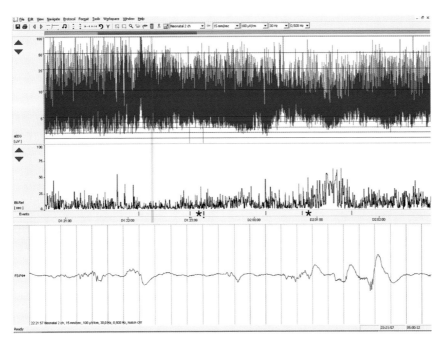

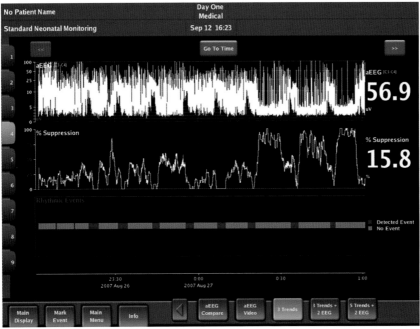

Figure 2.17 (a) This figure shows increased IBI in an extremely preterm infant, born at 22 weeks' gestation, who received morphine during mechanical ventilation. This infant received two bolus doses of morphine, the first one at time 23:10 and the second at 00:45 (asterisks). At 01:30 a continuous infusion of morphine was started. The time is shown below the IBI as D1 (day 1):hh:mm. Care procedures were performed at time 22:15 and 00:15 (suctioning of the endotracheal tube). The first dose of morphine did not affect the IBI but the second dose resulted in a transient increase in IBI. The 25 s of EEG at the bottom were recorded at time 22:21, 11 minutes after the first dose of morphine.

(b) This figure shows increasing discontinuity in the aEEG, here also displayed with a trend showing percentage of suppression, during a 2-h recording of an infant with repetitive seizures on a discontinuous background. The progressive depression of the electrocortical background is visible in the aEEG at the end of the recording, but difficult to estimate before. Figure and videoclip courtesy of Damon Lees and Gary Trapuzzano.

Effect of surfactant administration

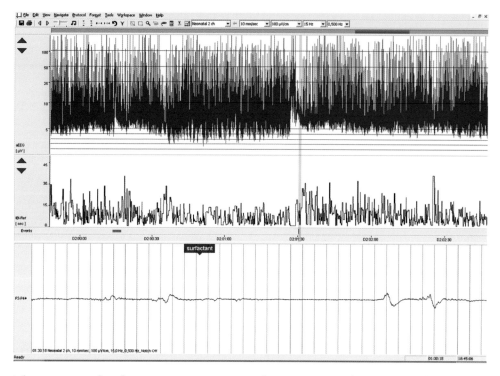

Figure 2.18 Administration of surfactant may sometimes result in a transient depression of electrocortical activity. The reason for this is not known.[51] This infant, born at 24 gestational weeks, received a second dose of surfactant (light blue vertical line through aEEG). The resulting mild decrease in activity is seen in the aEEG with both decreasing burst rate and increasing IBI. The 25 s of EEG below shows the rather inactive background, with superimposed fast low-amplitude activity from the high-frequency ventilation.

3

Pitfalls and caveats

In this chapter we will discuss and illustrate some pitfalls and caveats encountered during aEEG monitoring in the NICU. The development of new digital monitors, allowing access to the original EEG, has been associated with great improvements, since inspection of the EEG signal is by far the best way of disclosing extracerebral artifact sources as possible causes of unexpected changes in the aEEG trend patterns (see Figure 1.7). As for all EEG recording, careful control of electrode impedance is important in order to avoid pick-up of artifacts. Most aEEG recording equipment provides tools for continuous surveillance of signal quality and impedance. Staff taking care of the patient should be instructed how to detect and interpret high impedances and when to suspect a loose electrode (Figure 3.1).

Care procedures often produce movement artifacts that cause a sudden shift in the aEEG trace, which is usually easily identified in the original EEG signal (Figure 3.2). In premature infants and sick term infants with discontinuous EEG activity such procedures may cause an arousal, and a transient period of continuous EEG with a sudden increase in the minimum level of the aEEG trace, which is sometimes mistaken for a solitary period of seizure activity. In more healthy term infants with a continuous normal voltage (CNV) pattern, arousing stimuli cause a transient increase in low-amplitude high-frequency EEG components, and a decrease in low-frequency components (see Figure 1.1b). Due to the filter properties of the aEEG recording this does not always produce a discernible shift in the aEEG trace. This is presumably one reason why the presence or absence of arousal responses has not been associated with

prognosis in several aEEG studies. Handling of the infant, as well as administration of drugs, should always be marked on the recording. Sometimes frequent care procedures seem to cause a deterioration in a discontinuous pattern in extremely preterm infants; the reason for this is not known, but adverse reactions to cluster care have been described in other studies.[56] Repeated gasping or other repeated motor activity may be misinterpreted as a discontinuous EEG pattern in infants with very poor and depressed EEG background, and inspection of the original EEG does not always solve this interpretational problem. Visual inspection of the infant in relation to the ongoing aEEG/EEG changes may solve the problem, as may administration of a muscle relaxant to mechanically ventilated infants in these relatively rare situations (see Figure 3.3).

As discussed in Chapter 2, great emphasis is given to the minimum amplitude level of the aEEG trace, for evaluation of both continuous and discontinuous EEG patterns. The amplitude of the electrocortical activity is important, but this measure must be handled with caution as the EEG signal may be affected by a number of factors. Electrode positions during clinical EEG monitoring may have to be adjusted due to, e.g., skin lacerations after vacuum extraction and cephalic hematoma. Classification according to amplitude requires a standard interelectrode distance, as a reduction of this distance may cause a reduction in amplitude (Figures 3.4–3.6). Deviations from standard recording derivations may also modify the recorded amplitude levels. Furthermore, scalp edema may reduce the EEG signal by electric shunting. In two-channel bipolar recordings asymmetric interelectrode distances or an asymmetric scalp edema after vacuum extraction may produce an artificial asymmetry. Problems related to asymmetries or focal abnormalities should always be addressed by a full EEG recording.

The NICU is a very EEG 'unfriendly' environment with several electrical and mechanical sources of artifacts. High-frequency ventilation usually adds to the input signal with an upward shift of the baseline. In the new aEEG equipment this is usually revealed by a low-amplitude monorhythmic EEG signal with the same frequency as the high-frequency ventilation (Figure 3.7).

A shift in head position, leading to mechanical contact between the electrodes and the pillow/bedding, may cause sudden changes in the aEEG background when high-frequency ventilation and other mechanical artifacts interfere with the recording (Figure 3.8). Unexplained upward shifts of the baseline level in records expected to be flat or suppression burst is a relatively common finding. Sometimes the explanation is revealed in the original EEG record as ECG or pulsative mechanical movements (Figure 3.9). When in doubt, a full EEG recording and consultation with a clinical neurophysiologist is recommended.

SUMMARY

- The aEEG is sensitive to interference from various artifact sources from surrounding electronic equipment and from the infant such as muscle activity, movements, high-frequency ventilation, and ECG.

- The input impedance of the recording electrodes should be kept <5 kΩ. Staff taking care of the patient should be instructed to detect a loose electrode or high electrode impedance.

- Frequent clinical notes in the recording system on care procedures and medication will facilitate later interpretation.

- Do not apply needle electrodes above fontanelles or sutures.

- Do not apply electrodes over cephalic hematoma or other local abnormalities on the skull.

- Do not position electrodes in direct contact with bedding.

- At least one full conventional EEG should be performed in most infants with aEEG monitoring.

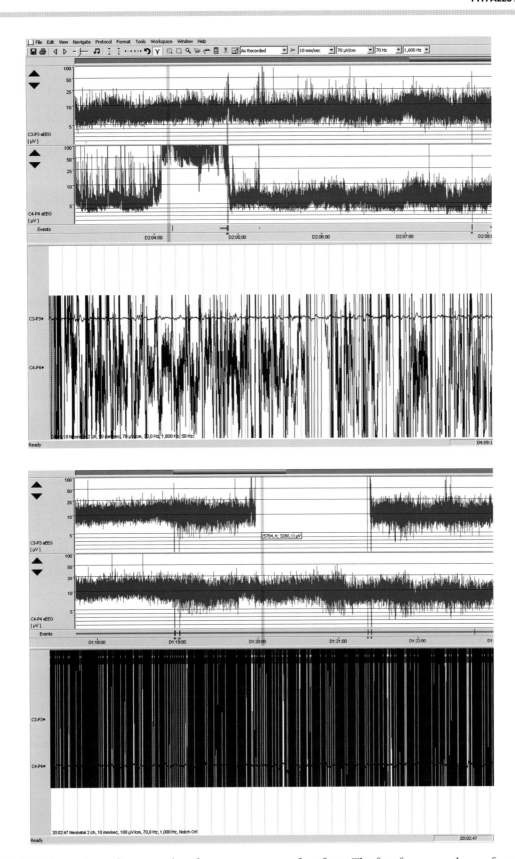

Figure 3.1 This figure shows five examples of common sources of artifacts. The first four examples are from NicoletOne recordings, but these artifacts appear very similar also in the other EEG monitors. Panels (a) to (d) show bilateral two-channel aEEG/EEG recordings from C3–P3 and C4–P4: (a) poor electrode on the right side; (b) loose electrode on the left side;

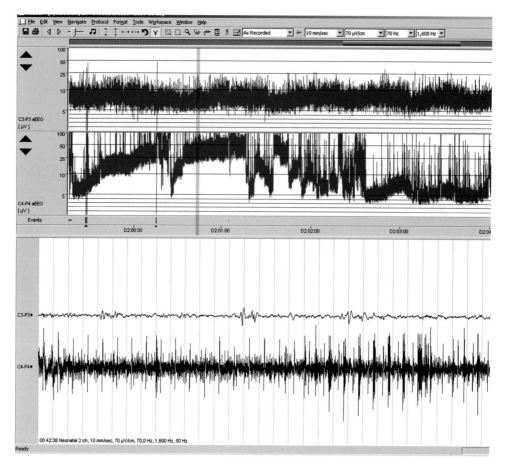

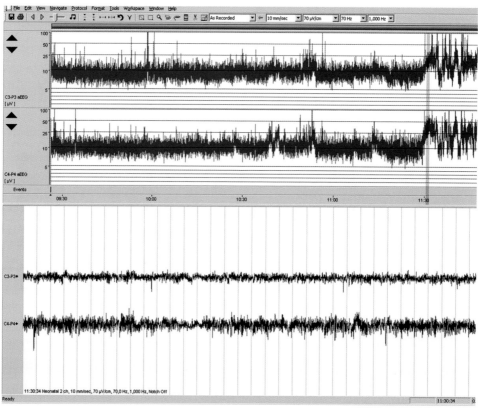

Figure 3.1 *continued*

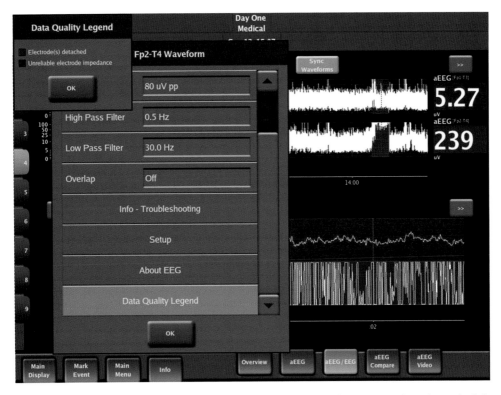

Figure 3.1 *opposite and above* (c) baseline shift on the right side due to muscle activity; (d) at the end of this trace there is bilateral upward deflection of the aEEG which could be mistaken for seizures but is caused by muscle activity; (e) loose electrode on the right side (Fp2–T4) and automated detection of electrode failure.

Transient changes during caregiving

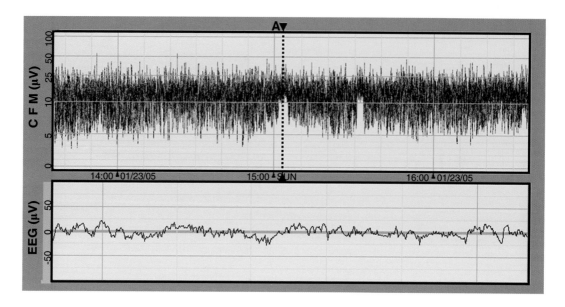

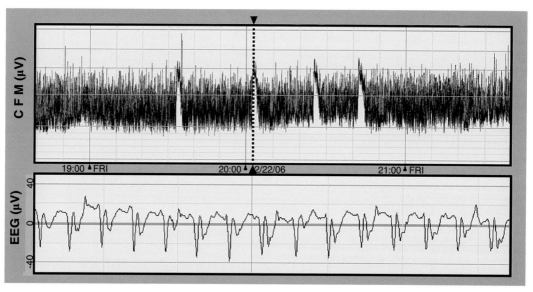

Figure 3.2 (a) This infant with HIE (see Figure 5.5 for full story) had a slightly discontinuous background pattern. Concomitant with a caregiving procedure (marker A), and representing arousal due to handling, a transient increase in the minimum amplitude of the aEEG can be seen. The second rise in activity occurs 30 min later; there are no clinical notes here but it is likely that this was also caused by caregiving since no ictal activity was seen in the original EEG. With the gray scale, one would expect an increase of both the lower and upper margin of the trace, and a 'cap' during the transient increase in the minimum aEEG amplitude, in case of an ictal discharge. This is illustrated by the second panel (b), from another infant with HIE. The original EEG helped to make a distinction between the artifact and the ictal discharge, which was clearly confirmed in the second example.

Effect of care in an extremely preterm infant

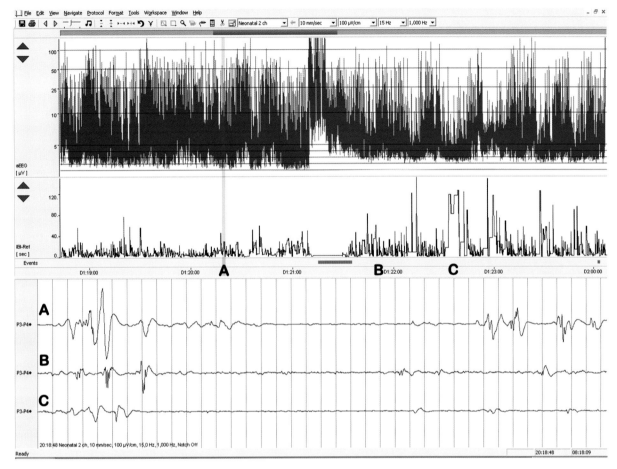

Figure 3.3 This is a 6-h recording of an extremely preterm infant, born at 24 gestational weeks, who had a care procedure (green horizontal line in the figure) performed at the age of 12 hours. The aEEG clearly shows the increased depression of activity after this procedure, which is also reflected as an increase in the IBI trend. The EEG samples below show 25 s of discontinuous EEG before (A) and after (B and C) the care procedure. There is no obvious change in the EEG, instead the trend measures aEEG/IBI can better display the deterioration in the background activity.

Effect of gasping

HIE III

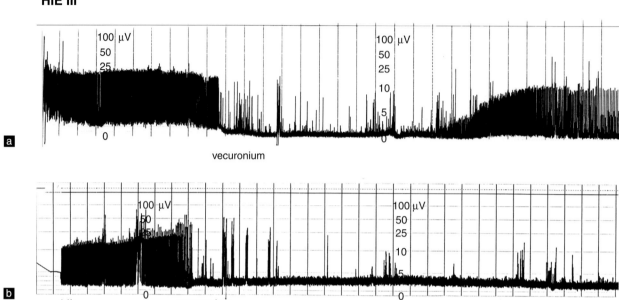

Figure 3.4 (a) This aEEG tracing is from a full-term infant with severe HIE. The infant was continuously gasping on the ventilator. The initial aEEG can easily be misinterpreted as a BS pattern. However, following a loading dose of vecuronium, a muscle relaxant, the aEEG became flat and revealed the true state of cerebral function in this infant. After about 2 h, the effect of the muscle-paralyzing agent was wearing off. The gasping started again, and in the aEEG again a BS-like background was seen. The impedance was low all the time.

(b) The lower tracing from another severely asphyxiated infant is very similar except that a continuous infusion of vecuronium was given. There was no return of gasping and the aEEG remained flat.

Both examples were reproduced from the previous edition of the aEEG Atlas.[57]

Artifacts due to gasping are rare, but should be excluded when severely brain-injured infants on mechanical ventilation are gasping and the aEEG shows a BS-like pattern. The original EEG is helpful, but not always conclusive.

Effect of incorrect electrode positioning

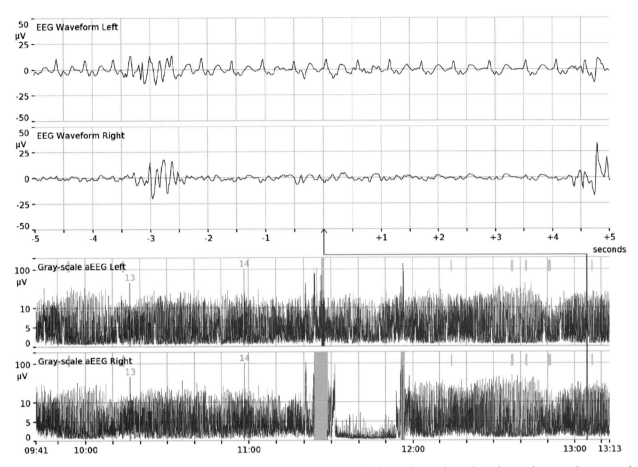

Figure 3.5 In this full-term infant with a metabolic disorder a needle electrode on the right side was loose and reinserted (red block on the right side at time 11:30). Following the repositioning, a flattening of the recording was seen. The electrodes were found to be very near to each other; when reapplied at an increased distance the background pattern was comparable to before the disconnection of the electrode. During the recording brief ictal discharges are seen on the left side, as shown by the EEG at time 13:04, and also as indicated by the seizure detection alerts (orange markers).

Recording channels and aEEG amplitudes

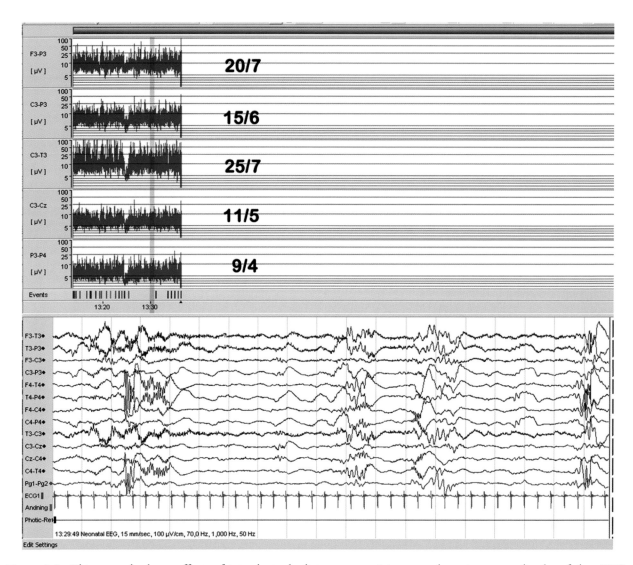

Figure 3.6 This example shows effects of interelectrode distances on minimum and maximum amplitudes of the aEEG. The EEG was recorded in a preterm baby (GA 31 weeks) who was born by emergency Cesarean section due to placental abruption. Apgar scores were 1/2/7. The infant developed severe respiratory distress syndrome (RDS) and initially required high-frequency ventilation, but could be extubated on day 3. The cranial ultrasound showed small bilateral subependymal hemorrhages (IVH 1). The baby survived and was discharged to a local hospital in apparently good health.

The short aEEG traces were created from the EEG, the channels are above: F3–P3; C3–P3; C3–T3; C3–Cz; P3–P4. The average maximum and minimum amplitude values for the aEEG epochs are indicated in the figure. The proximity between the electrodes for C3–Cz and P3–P4, respectively, is demonstrated by their relatively lower amplitudes.

Effect of high-frequency ventilation

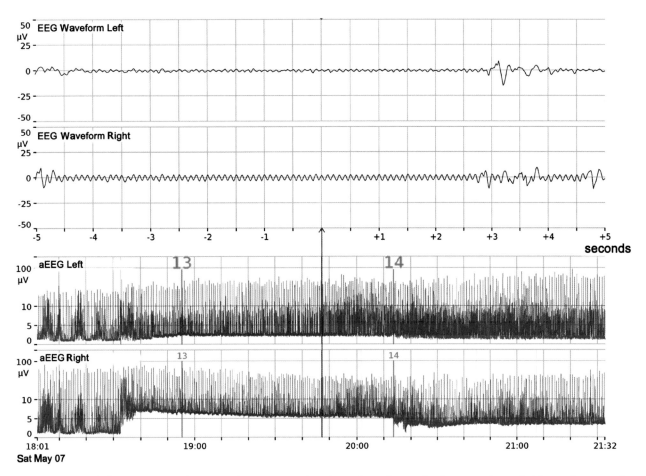

Figure 3.7 High-frequency ventilation is often associated with artifacts that make the aEEG less reliable, as shown in this full-term infant with severe HIE. In the beginning of the aEEG recording there is a sudden elevation of the lower margin on the right side, which is probably due to the baby turning to the right, allowing the electrodes to be in contact with the bedding, although this is not marked. The original EEG at time 19:47 shows fast rhythmic 10 Hz activity of low voltage, i.e. a high-frequency ventilation artifact which should not be confused with ictal activity. Suctioning in the endotracheal tube is done at marker 13. At marker 14 the head is turned to the midline position, resulting in a downward shift of the baseline level on the right side. This drift of the baseline often occurs when there is contact between the electrode and the bedding when an infant is on high-frequency ventilation.

Effect of electrode and head position

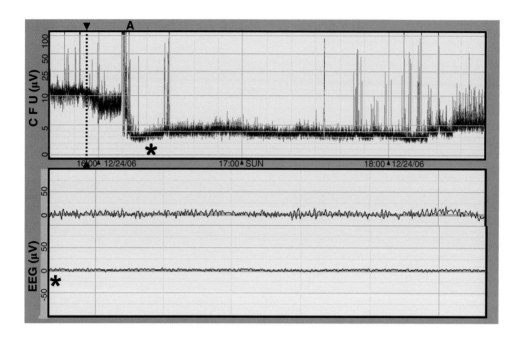

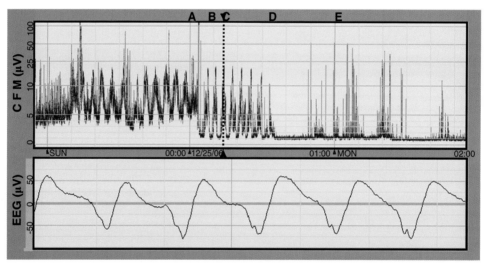

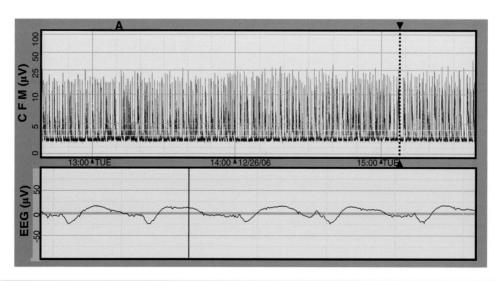

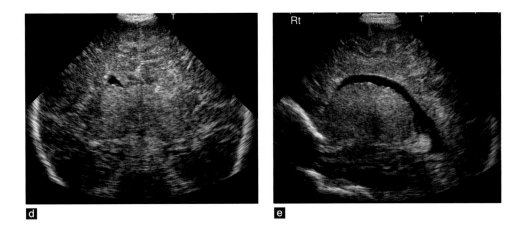

d

e

Figure 3.8 *opposite and above* This male infant was born at full term in a planned home delivery which was complicated by a placental abruption. He was resuscitated and started to show some spontaneous breathing after 45 minutes. The first capillary blood gas showed a pH of 6.93 with a base excess of –25 mmol/l. On arrival to the NICU he was restless and making a lot of abnormal rowing movements. He required ventilatory support, but intensive care was later withdrawn in view of the poor prognosis.

Cranial ultrasound showed a diffusely echogenic brain with compression of the left lateral ventricle and increased echogenicity of the right thalamus in particular. The child was too unstable to be transported to the MR unit.

On admission the aEEG registration was started. The initial part of the recording (panel a) showed a pattern that looked continuous and not in agreement with the condition of the infant, who had abundant abnormal motor activity. The corresponding original EEG showed high-frequency muscular activity artifacts, and inspection of the electrodes showed that they were placed just above the ears at the level of the temporal muscles. Following repositioning of the needle electrodes (A), the muscle artifact resolved and the trace now revealed a flat background pattern which was also confirmed by an inactive EEG. At 12 h he developed repetitive seizures on a very suppressed background recording (panel b). Note the effect of head turning on the background pattern (A), the absent effect of vecuronium (B), the continuing seizures and further depression of background activity following midazolam (C), and the flat trace following lidocaine bolus (D) and infusion (E). However, seizures recurred after 48 h, and panel c shows a subclinical status epilepticus on an inactive background. This pattern could easily have been misinterpreted as a BS pattern, but the original EEG shows clear sharp and slow-wave complexes (see also videoclip).

This case illustrates the effect of the position of the electrodes and also the effect of the position of the head on the amplitude of the aEEG trace. It is also not uncommon to see that, following a prolonged period of a flat background, recovery can be seen as development of a BS pattern with a superimposed SE.

Baseline drift due to ECG artifact

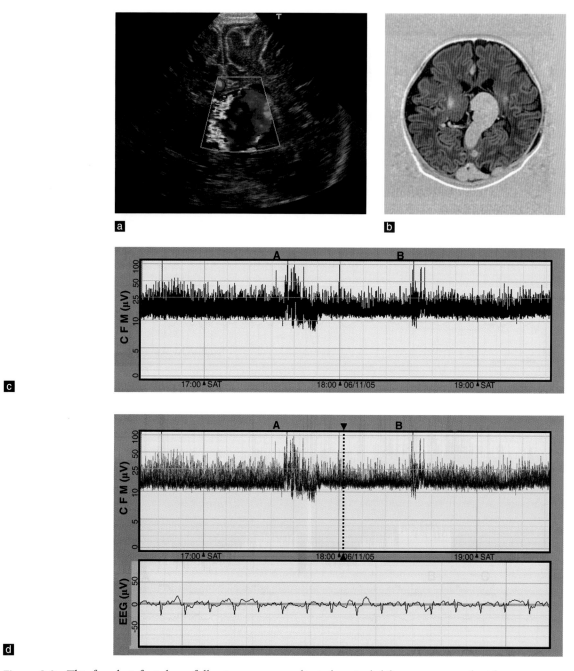

Figure 3.9 This female infant, born following an uncomplicated vaginal delivery, presented with symptoms suggestive of heart failure on day 5. An ultrasound of the heart did not show any structural abnormalities. However, a murmur was heard over the anterior fontanelle and a vein of Galen malformation was diagnosed.

Cranial ultrasound with Doppler flow measurement (a) and MRI (T1 weighted inversion recovery sequence) (b) diagnosed a large vein of Galen malformation.

As clinical seizures were suspected, an aEEG recording was initiated. The aEEG showed an apparently normal background pattern, although it was noted that the lower margin was not showing any variability (c). Using the gray scale (d), it was easier to appreciate the abnormal background pattern, with the darker band of activity weighted at the lower part of the tracing suggesting an elevated BS pattern. The original EEG mainly showed ECG artifacts, which was the reason for the drift of the baseline. A standard EEG performed simultaneously confirmed the presence of ECG artifacts superimposed on a discontinuous background pattern.

4

Seizures

Early detection of epileptic seizures in high-risk infants and evaluation of antiepileptic treatment in infants with diagnosed seizures are two important indications for continuous EEG monitoring in newborn infants.

Epileptic syndromes are rare in the neonatal period and most seizures are 'reactive', i.e. they appear during or after insults that include disturbed cerebral oxygenation, blood flow, or metabolism. Consequently, the most common etiologies of neonatal seizures include hypoxic–ischemic or hemorrhagic brain injury, hypoglycemia and metabolic diseases, severe infections such as sepsis and meningitis, congenital malformations, and maternal drug abuse. Pyridoxine-dependent seizures are rare; they may mimic hypoxic–ischemic encephalopathy, and as such they are probably underdiagnosed.[58] Other rare causes of neonatal seizures include benign familial neonatal-infantile seizures due to ion-channel mutations (potassium and sodium), and 'fifth-day seizures', which are idiopathic seizures that were more common one to two decades ago.[59–61]

INCIDENCE

The incidence of neonatal seizures varies between different studies due to differences in study populations, time periods, and criteria for diagnosing the seizures. Some studies include infants with clinically suspected seizures, while other studies required EEG-verified seizures, which will lower the incidence since only around 70% of clinically suspected seizures could be verified by EEG.[62] More recent data indicate that around 1–2 infants per 1000 live born are diagnosed with seizures, with a 5- to 10-fold increased risk in preterm infants.[63,64]

Seizures are, of course, more common in NICU populations, and even among them the incidence will vary according to the specific study population and diagnostic criteria. A combined approach for diagnosing seizures which included EEG and aEEG monitoring of high-risk infants resulted in a seizure incidence of 4.5%.[65] If selected high-risk populations, e.g. infants after cardiac surgery, are evaluated with continuous EEG monitoring, between 10 and 20% will be diagnosed with seizures.[66,67] Seizures, mainly subclinical, are also common in preterm infants developing peri/intraventricular hemorrhages. Studies from the 1980s and early 1990s using continuous EEG or aEEG showed that around 65–75% of preterm infants with intraventricular hemorrhages (IVH) developed seizures.[34,37,68] The overall incidence of IVH in preterm infants has decreased and there are no current figures on seizure prevalence in these infants.

Certain groups of infants in the NICU are at higher risk for developing seizures than others. Abnormal EEG background activity is an indicator of increased risk for seizures,[69] but there are no reliable clinical markers that identify the individual infants with the highest risks for seizures.[70] We therefore suggest the following indications for continuous EEG monitoring in order to enhance early identification of seizures:

- Perinatal asphyxia and hypoxic–ischemic encephalopathy;

- Infants with clinically suspected seizures;

- Severely ill infants (RDS, sepsis) who require mechanical ventilation and/or inotropes;

- Infants with meningitis, unspecified encephalopathy, or cerebral malformations;

- Infants with severe cardiac malformations or congenital diaphragmatic hernia;

- Infants with severe hypoglycemia or metabolic disease;

- Infants requiring ECMO treatment;

- Infants who receive paralyzing agents while being ventilated.

DIAGNOSING SEIZURES

Clinical identification

Neonatal seizures can be difficult to recognize since clinical symptoms may be subtle or entirely absent.[71,72] Also, when infants demonstrate clinically suspected seizures, it is not uncommon that these are not accompanied by corresponding electrographic seizure activity, as shown by Mizrahi and Kellaway using EEG video monitoring.[73] Clinical seizures can be classified as being either subtle, clonic, or tonic, and may be either focal, multifocal, or generalized.[74] In the current Atlas we have not reported detailed descriptions of seizure semiology (clinical seizure appearance) since a large number of seizures are often seen in continuous monitoring and the clinical expression may vary. When identified, the various clinical seizure types (subtle, clonic, tonic, myoclonic) seem to be similarly distributed in preterm infants above 30 weeks and term infants, while subclinical seizures are more common in extremely preterm infants.[75]

Neonatal seizures are often classified as being either electroclinical, i.e. electrographic changes with clinical symptoms, or electrographic, i.e. 'occult' or clinically silent. Newborn infants often display a mixture of electroclinical and electrographic seizure types, although the majority of seizures are clinically silent. Electroclinical 'uncoupling' is common, i.e. the clinical seizures cease while electrographic (subclinical) seizures persist after administration of antiepileptic drugs.[67,71,72,75–81]

In conclusion, clinical identification of seizures by clinical observation alone is unreliable in newborn infants. All infants with clinically suspected seizures should have a standard EEG recorded and EEG monitoring initiated as soon as possible in order to correctly diagnose electrographic seizure activity. Electroclinical 'uncoupling' after administration of antiepileptic medications is an important reason for using continuous EEG monitoring in infants with diagnosed seizures.

Electrographic identification

A seizure pattern in the EEG is characterized by repetitive, stereotyped waveforms (spikes, sharp waves, spike–slow-wave complexes, rhythmic theta or delta activity without sharp components) with a definite onset, peak, and end (crescendo-decrescendo appearance). There are no specific criteria as regards minimum duration of a seizure, although 10 s has been a criterion in many studies. Briefer runs of repetitive waveforms, often called epileptiform activity, are not uncommon in ill newborns. It is possible that shorter periods of repetitive activity, 5–10 s, should also be assessed as seizures since this type of activity has been associated with adverse neurologic sequelae.[82] Status epilepticus is often defined as continuously ongoing ictal activity or recurrent seizures of at least 30 minutes' duration, or more than 50% of the EEG recording time.

The duration of an individual seizure is usually quite short. Clancy and Legido[83] estimated that most neonatal seizures have a duration of less than 1 minute, while Scher et al estimated the average seizure duration to 5 minutes in term infants and 2 minutes in preterm infants.[84] The slightly diverging results could probably be explained by differences in the study populations; 87% of the infants in the study by Clancy and Legido received antiepileptic treatment, as compared to only 50% in the study by Scher et al.

The reason why seizures can be easily identified in the aEEG by pattern recognition is due to the increase and the decrease of EEG waveform frequencies and amplitudes. A seizure will result in a transient rise in the aEEG amplitude, maximum and minimum border, or sometimes only the minimum border (Figure 4.1a). Rarely, a seizure may also result in a transient decrease in the aEEG, due to an ictal flattening of the EEG activity (Figure 4.1b). Similar patterns have also been seen in infants with hypsarrhythmia and infantile spasms where seizures are associated with lower amplitude desynchronization of the high-voltage EEG background.[57] Continuously ongoing spiking, e.g. periodic lateralized or bilateral epileptiform discharges (PLEDs, BIPLEDs), may not be possible to identify in the aEEG since they are not associated with a transient change in the overall electrocortical background activity. However, their presence can sometimes be suspected in the aEEG when a continuously very high-voltage pattern is present, and they can, of course, be seen in the original EEG.

It is not uncommon that a few brief seizures appear during long-term routine EEG monitoring of infants during intensive care; sometimes repeated seizures can be seen, and in some infants status epilepticus is present (often subclinical).[85] The different density of seizures appearing during EEG monitoring constituted the rationale for our suggested classification/characterization of seizure patterns in the aEEG (see examples with corresponding EEGs in Figures 4.1a–f).[44] However, the aEEG does not give information about individual EEG waveforms or their topographic distribution during the seizures (Figure 4.3).

Optimal number of electrodes

The number of electrodes necessary for optimal identification and treatment of neonatal seizures is not known. Most seizures in newborn infants seem to start in the temporal and central areas.[86] Preterm infants usually have a regional onset of seizures, while the onset in full-term infants often is more focal. Consequently, when using EEG monitoring with a reduced number of electrodes, i.e. one or two channels, clinicians must be aware that not all electrographic seizure activity will be detected/shown. A reduction from 12 to 4 EEG electrodes in 32 neonates with seizures resulted in underestimation of the number of seizures in 19 infants, and two infants with seizures were not identified.[87] Comparable figures were obtained by Tekgul et al: reducing the number of EEG electrodes from 19 to 9 resulted in a significantly lower (only 166/187) number of identified seizures and one infant, out of 31, with seizures was not identified.[88]

Recently published data show that a single-channel EEG derived from two electrodes (P3–P4 or C3–C4) identifies 80–90% of infants with seizures.[80,89] The precision of the aEEG in diagnosing seizures without display of the original EEG is lower. In a study comparing seizure detection in a single-channel aEEG versus a full EEG, 851 seizures were identified in 125 EEG recordings from 121 neonates. However, only 26% of seizures and 40% of infants were identified by the aEEG when there was no display of the EEG. The single-channel EEG from C3–C4 identified 78% of seizures and 94% of infants with seizures, in spite of relatively short EEG recordings (23–145 minutes).[89] The explanation for the low seizure recognition in the aEEG without display of the EEG is the overall short duration of neonatal seizures which renders them impossible to identify in the very time-compressed display of the aEEG, also shown by several examples in this Atlas. This was also demonstrated by an earlier study which compared aEEG with EEG in single- or five-channel recordings (total duration 226.8 h). Seizures developed in 6 out of 10 infants with single-channel aEEG/EEG and in four of the five infants with five-channel recordings. Altogether five infants developed status epilepticus, which was detected by the single-channel aEEG from P3–P4. However, only 15 of 48 EEG-verified single seizures could be detected in the aEEG (without display of the EEG); this, in turn, corresponded to only four clinically recognized seizures.[90] The seizures that were not detectable by the aEEG, but were identified by the EEG, were all of short duration (5–30 s). Similar results for seizure detection with the aEEG alone or in combination with EEG were also obtained in a study of infants with hypoxic–ischemic encephalopathy. Furthermore, the duration of electrical seizure activity observed on the two-channel bedside aEEG monitor strongly correlated with the duration of the seizures observed on the conventional EEG.[91]

In theory, two channels (one over each hemisphere) would identify more seizures than one channel (bilateral). However, preliminary data do not support this; instead, one channel seems to be as efficient as two channels for detecting seizures.[92] Furthermore, with a five-channel EEG it was shown that all seizure activity (>30 s) was detectable in the single-channel EEG recording derived from P3–P4 locations.[90] Also focal EEG seizure activity produces voltage gradients over the skull, which can often be picked up with bipolar leads provided that a large enough distance between the recording electrodes is used, such as with the biparietal (P3–P4) or bilateral fronto-parietal (F3–P3, F4–P4) montages.

Moderate hypothermia is increasingly used as a neuroprotective intervention after severe birth asphyxia. Although this has currently not been evaluated in newborn infants, experimental data suggest that cooling is associated with lower seizure amplitudes.[93] If seizures in cooled newborn infants are also of lower amplitudes, they might be more difficult to identify in the aEEG/EEG monitoring, and measures should be taken to avoid too short interelectrode distances.

Automated detection of seizures

The new digital EEG monitors with simultaneous display of EEG and EEG trends enhance the possibilities for accurate interpretation and diagnosis of epileptic seizure activity. However, as with any new technology, it is important to understand its benefits and limitations before relying on it for decisions related to patient care.

Algorithms have been created for automated seizure detection in neonatal EEG and aEEG, some of which have been published.[94–96] However, the variable waveforms and appearances of neonatal seizures constitute a challenge for automated seizure detection systems which require high precision, i.e. high sensitivity and specificity with a low number of false-positive alarms. A majority of the new EEG monitors have implemented seizure detection algorithms for 'alerts' or 'event detection' of neonatal seizures. Although some of these systems may show very high sensitivities and low false detection rates, it is important to understand that the precision is not 100%. They can therefore only serve as an 'aid' for the neonatal staff who still have to evaluate both the aEEG patterns and the original EEGs unless departments of neurology or neurophysiology provide this service 24 h per day, 7 days per week.

Other trends than the aEEG can also be used in order to facilitate identification of seizures. This has not been formally evaluated, but we have found displays including density spectral array (DSA) to be helpful to detect seizures, (see Figures 1.11 and 4.4a and b).

TREATMENT OF NEONATAL SEIZURES

It is outside the scope of this Atlas to discuss treatment of neonatal seizures, whether they are clinical or subclinical, single or repetitive. Antiepileptic drugs and indications for when they should be administered have been the focus of long-term discussions during the last decades. Long-term prophylactic treatment in infants presenting seizures in the neonatal period may not be necessary in a majority of cases.[65,97]

Although not investigated in any controlled study, two studies using aEEG monitoring for diagnosing and treating subclinical seizures in newborns appear to have a lower risk for postneonatal epilepsy than comparable NICU populations, even with a median duration of antiepileptic treatment as short as 4.5 days.[65,98]

PROGNOSIS

Seizures in newborn infants are associated with mortality, and risk for postneonatal epilepsy and adverse neurodevelopmental outcome in survivors. Several factors influence the long-term prognosis, including the etiology of the seizures, the maturity of the infant, and the seizure 'burden'. Infants with intractable seizures, and seizures associated with severely abnormal EEG background, have the worst outcomes.[75,99,100] Subclinical seizures and brief rhythmic discharges have also been reported to be associated with a poor outcome.[82,101]

SUMMARY

- A main indication for (a)EEG monitoring is clinical surveillance of 'high-risk' infants.

- Neonatal seizures are often subtle or subclinical.

- EEG monitoring is clearly superior to clinical signs for identification of neonatal seizures.

- The limited number of electrodes makes the aEEG method easy to use for clinical routine monitoring in the NICU.

- Continuous EEG monitoring with a reduced number of electrodes detects around 80% of seizures, and at least 90% of infants with seizures.

- A full standard EEG should be recorded in all infants early during the monitoring, and repeated as required.

- Close collaboration between the NICU and departments of neurology and/or clinical neurophysiology increases the chances for optimal use of EEG monitoring.

Different types of aEEG seizure patterns

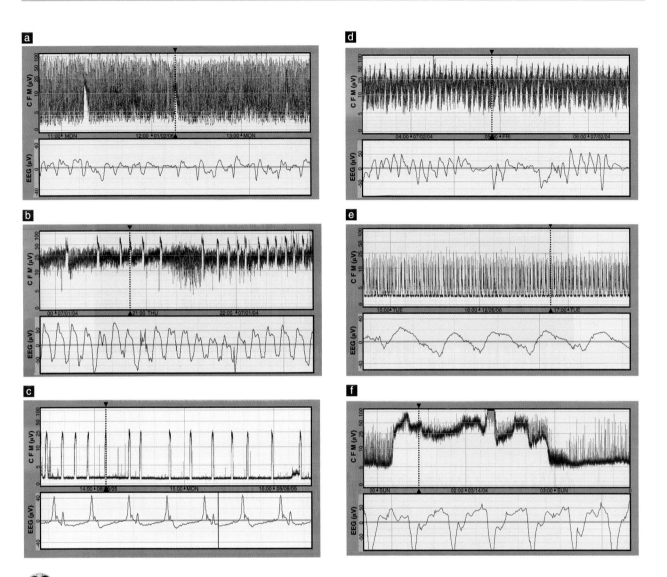

Figure 4.1 This figure shows different types of seizure patterns in the aEEG. The 6 s of EEG below the aEEG tracings correspond to the dotted vertical lines in the aEEGs, videoclips are available for all six panels.

(a) Two single seizures on a discontinuous background. The seizures appear with a 1-h interval; each one can be seen as a transient rise of the lower margin. The original EEG shows slightly irregular 2–3 Hz spike-wave complexes.

(b) Repetitive seizures on a CNV background pattern. All seizures are seen as transient rises of both the lower and upper margins of the aEEG. The corresponding EEG below shows rhythmic spike-wave complexes of 3 Hz.

(c) Repetitive seizures arising on an inactive (isoelectric) background. The EEG during the seizures shows slow (0.7 Hz) polyspike-wave complexes.

(d) Status epilepticus ('saw-tooth pattern') of at least 3 hours' duration (i.e. the whole screen) on a potentially good electrocortical background.

(e) This example also shows status epilepticus but on a very suppressed background. The status epilepticus could easily be mistaken for a BS pattern. The original EEG shows 0.7 Hz slow waves without clear spikes but with superimposed ECG artifacts.

(f) Status epilepticus with continuously ongoing seizure activity for almost 2 h. During this time the baseline is continuously raised; before and after this a BS pattern with sparse burst density is seen. If only the aEEG is evaluated during the status epilepticus it could easily be mistaken for CNV, but the EEG below reveals the true epileptic nature of this change in the aEEG background. The corresponding EEG shows slow rhythmical spike-wave complexes at around 1 Hz.

Different types of aEEG seizure patterns

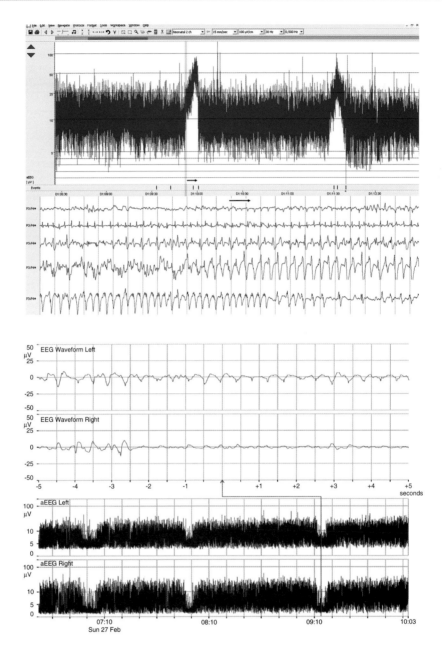

Figure 4.2 (a) This figure shows 4 h of aEEG from a postoperative recording in an infant after cardiac surgery. Altogether five subclinical seizures were noted during the first 24 postoperative hours; two of them are shown here. The five 25-s epochs of EEG are taken from the first seizure (short black arrow on aEEG), which has a duration of 10 min, and shows how the seizures start (long black arrow on the uppermost EEG trace) and how the EEG frequencies and amplitudes gradually increase and then decrease during the seizure and the resulting transient change in the aEEG trace.

(b) This example also shows a full-term infant with congenital heart disease, with aEEG recording before surgery. The seizure pattern in the discontinuous aEEG shows three seizures where a decrease in amplitude rather than a rise is seen. These episodes were recognized as ictal discharges, seen as low voltage (<25 μV) spike-wave complexes at about 2 Hz, on the simultaneous original EEG. This seizure appearance is unusual, but has also been seen in a few infants with hypsarrhythmia where the seizure is represented by desynchronization which is of lower voltage than the abnormal high-voltage background.

These two examples are both recordings in cardiac patients, one pre- and the other postsurgery, showing the use in this group of infants, who usually have extensive monitoring of their cardiovascular system, but not routinely of their central nervous system.

Variable EEG and aEEG waveforms during (subclinical) status epilepticus

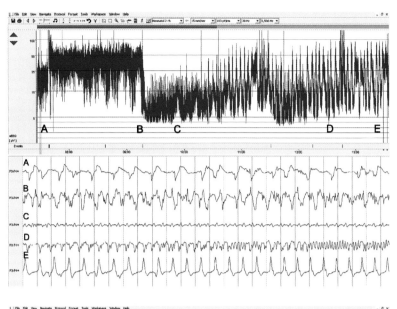

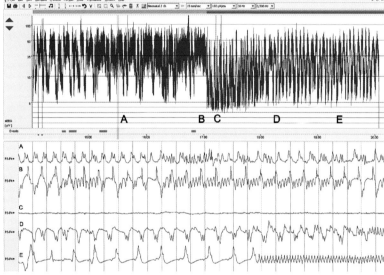

Figure 4.3 This infant with perinatal asphyxia was born at 41 gestational weeks; Apgar scores were 1/6/8, and the umbilical artery pH was 7.26. Clinical seizures started at 5 h, but they stopped after administration of diazepam. However, a subclinical status epilepticus continued for the following 48 h. Only on one occasion during this time period was a clinically suspected seizure observed. Several antiepileptic medications were administered, including phenobarbital, midazolam, lidocaine, fos-phenytoin, pyridoxine, and pentobarbital. The infant survived with epilepsy and severe cerebral palsy. The green horizontal lines denote care procedures.

The two panels of aEEG represent the first 12 (6+6) h after the infant's arrival in the regional NICU. The duration of the EEG samples below the aEEGs is 25 s. An electrographic status epilepticus is continuously ongoing with different types of waveforms. The various frequencies and amplitudes of the waveforms in the EEG are represented by the amplitude in the aEEG; this is especially evident in the upper panel trace C. The transient amplitude depression at B in both panels was due to administration of pentobarbital. Short periods (< 1 min) without seizure activity but with severely depressed background, mainly inactive, are present in the lower panel, and can be seen at C.

This case shows the variability in EEG waveforms during seizures, and how these waveforms can be seen as 'saw-tooth' patterns in the aEEG during status epilepticus. This case also shows an example of 'uncoupling', i.e. how clinical seizures may continue as subclinical for prolonged periods after administration of antiepileptic medications.

Status epilepticus that was not detected

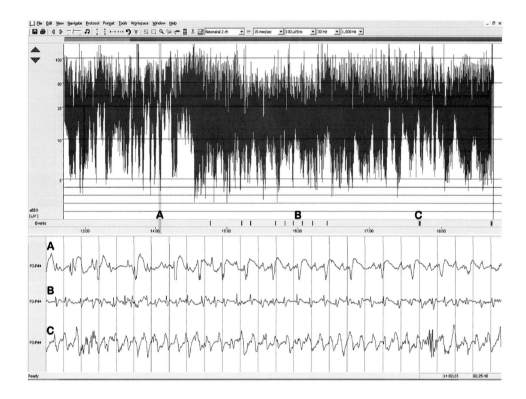

Figure 4.4 This twin infant, born at 32 weeks'gestation, was initially doing well but developed a respiratory syncytial (RS) virus infection at 4 weeks of age. The infection was associated with irritability and frequent apneas. A lumbar puncture did not show any abnormalities. The aEEG was initiated because of irritability. This infant was one of the first to be recorded with a new monitor showing simultaneous EEG and the neonatal staff was not used to this or the new aEEG display, and consequently did not notice the subclinical status epilepticus that was present for most of the 7 h of the recording (6 h shown here). Frequent clinical notes were performed: sleeping, crying, hiccups, apneas, etc. On one occasion a suspected seizure was noted (C). The infant survived and had follow-up until 3 years of age. During the first year of life the psychomotor development was slightly slower than that of the other twin, but later there was full catch-up.

This case shows the importance of teaching neonatal staff to evaluate the original EEG as well, and also the necessity of creating local standards for evaluation of EEG trend recordings.

Other EEG trends can assist in identification of seizures

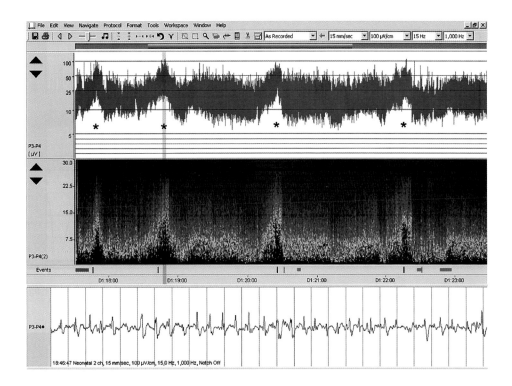

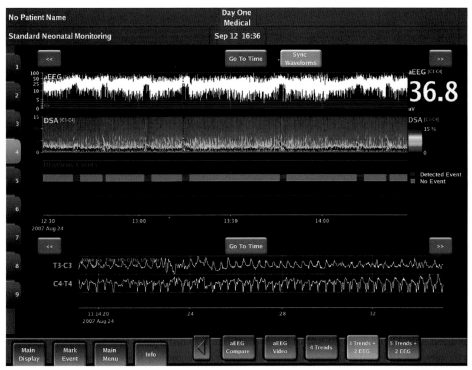

Figure 4.5 These two figures show how aEEG can be combined with other EEG trends, e.g. spectrogram/density spectral array (DSA), to enhance detection of neonatal seizures. The upper panel (a) shows aEEG and DSA during a 6-h recording with four seizures (asterisks) and 25 s of EEG from the second seizure (blue vertical line through the trends). The seizures are clearly seen as transient peaks of activity in both the aEEG and DSA. The lower panel (b) shows single-channel aEEG, DSA, and rhythmic event detection during a 2-h recording containing seven seizures. Below is 20 s of a two-channel EEG taken from the fourth seizure (dotted red vertical line through aEEG at time 13:15). Figure 4.5(b) provided courtesy of Damon Lees.

A preterm infant with myoclonic seizures

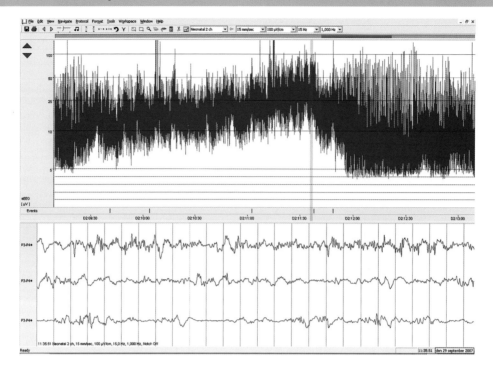

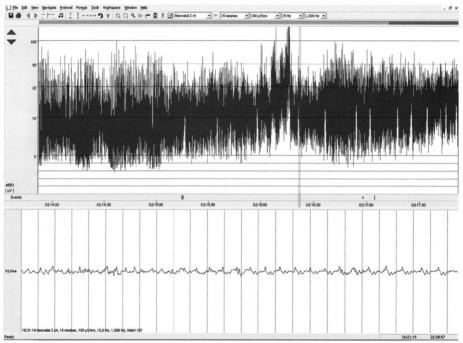

Figure 4.6 This male infant was the second child to a healthy mother. The pregnancy was normal until labor started at 33 week's gestation. Birthweight was 1950 g, and Apgar scores were 9, 10, and 10 at 1, 5, and 10 min, respectively. The amniotic fluid was meconium stained, and the arterial umbilical cord pH was 7.08 with a base excess of −12 mmol/l. Immediately after birth he was very distressed and agitated; he was lying in the opisthotonic position with stretched arms and fisted hands, and he was subsequently given thiopental and was intubated. He had suspected seizures on the aEEG/EEG and was given pyridoxine. A full standard EEG the following day showed BS but no seizures, and a new EEG on day 2 showed more continuous activity but still no seizures. He was extubated, and seemed to be well until 2 days later when he again developed clinical seizures (clonic seizures with apnea and eye blinking). An extensive investigation did not reveal any abnormalities, an MRI was considered normal. Several arterial lactate values were 3.5–5 mmol/l at the time when he also had clinical seizures. Seizures progressed and became more myclonic in spite of antiepileptic treatment with phenobarbital, diazepam, midazolam, thiopental, fos-phenytoin, lidocaine, clonazepam, topiramate, vigabatrin, levetiracetam, and with additional pyridoxin, thiamine, folic acid, vitamin B12, carnitine, biotin, and betamethasone. He seemed to respond temporarily to pyridoxine and thiamine and also to thiopental. Intensive care treatment was withdrawn after several weeks of intractable seizures.

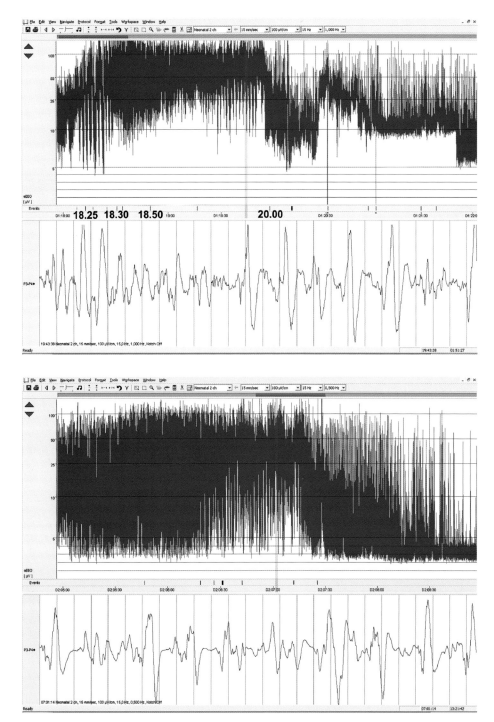

Figure 4.6 *opposite and above* The aEEGs above, each of 4 hours' duration, were recorded between days 5 and 7. (a) Response to pyridoxine; the upper EEG trace is taken just before pyridoxine (which was given right after the vertical blue line at around time 11:40) and the two lower EEG traces are taken a few minutes and 20 minutes later, respectively. Electrocortical background became transiently discontinuous. (b) Short seizures, accompanied by apneas, recurred within a few hours, as shown by the brief rises in the aEEG. At this time, the background activity had recovered and was continuous. (c) Intense electroclinical seizures developed again, and he received pyridoxine at time 18:25, midazolam at 18:30, and fos-phenytoin at 18:50 before he was intubated at 20:00 and then given thiopental and morphine, resulting in a decrease in the aEEG amplitude. New clinical seizures recurred 10 min later and more pentobarbital was given. (d) This panel shows the aEEG on day 7 and the EEG 15 min before a new loading dose of thiopental was given at time 07:15, resulting in severe background depression.

Seizure patterns that may be difficult to diagnose with the aEEG

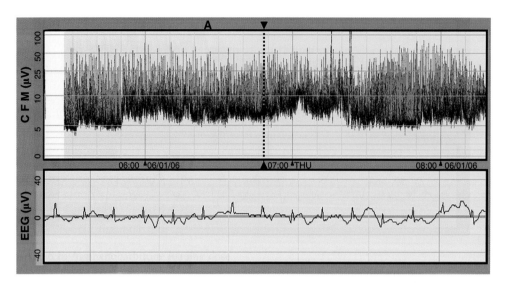

3h; A: tremors of the tongue.

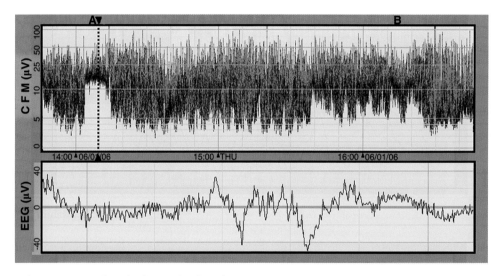

12h; A, care; B, phenobarbitone loading dose.

Figure 4.7 This female infant was born at home at 37 weeks' gestation with a birthweight of 2970 g. The Apgar scores were 3, 3, and 3 at 1, 5, and 10 min, respectively. She was taken to hospital where she was intubated before she was transferred to the regional level III NICU. Initially she had hypoglycemia (blood glucose 0.4 mmol/l) and metabolic acidosis with an arterial lactate of 19.9 mmol/l. She had aEEG monitoring which revealed repeated epileptic subclinical seizures (see below). Following the initial problems, she recovered well although she had a persisting low platelet count. Her clinical condition deteriorated again 10 days later, when she was readmitted and was diagnosed with a thrombus of the abdominal aorta. A laparotomy was performed and showed complete necrosis of almost the entire intestine, and intensive care was subsequently withdrawn.

(a) The aEEG was started at 3 h after birth, and showed a BS pattern with a lower margin above 5 μV, i.e. 'drift of the baseline' due to ECG artifact which can be seen in the original EEG with low-voltage 'spikes' with a frequency around 2 Hz corresponding to a heart rate of 120 beats/min. Note the scale of the EEG on the y-axis, which displays the low-amplitude ECG artifact in such a way that it can be mistaken for seizure activity. In the second panel (b), starting at 12 h of age, there is a period during care which could be mistaken for a discharge, without notation by the nurse or without the original EEG to review this period. A few hours later, repeated seizures can be seen as a 'saw-tooth pattern' in the aEEG (the epileptic nature verified by the original EEG), and phenobarbitone was given.

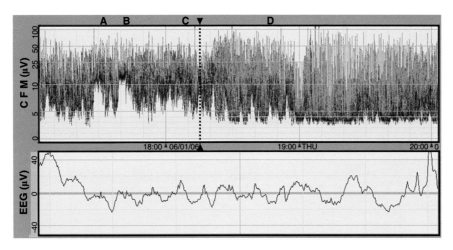

16h; A and B, care; C, ultrasound examination; D, midazolam.

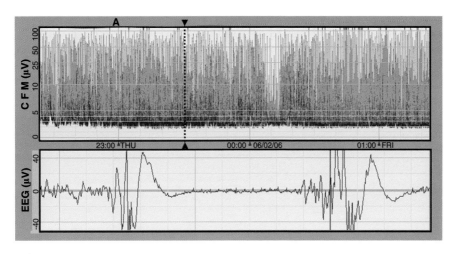

46h.

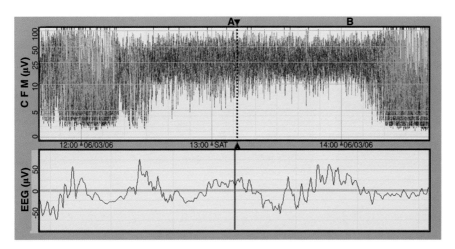

60h; A, start EEG recording; B, phenobarbitone loading dose.

Figure 4.7 *opposite and above*   The seizures were not controlled by phenobarbitone, and midazolam was given (D) in the third panel (c). The midazolam seems to control the seizures, but also changed the background from discontinuous to BS, which continued the following day (d). At 60 h (e) there is a sudden rise in the background amplitude which continues for almost 2 h. This change could be misinterpreted as improvement in the electrocortical background, but it was rather sudden and the original EEG showed repeated brief (3–5 s) periods of rhythmic 4–5 Hz activity.

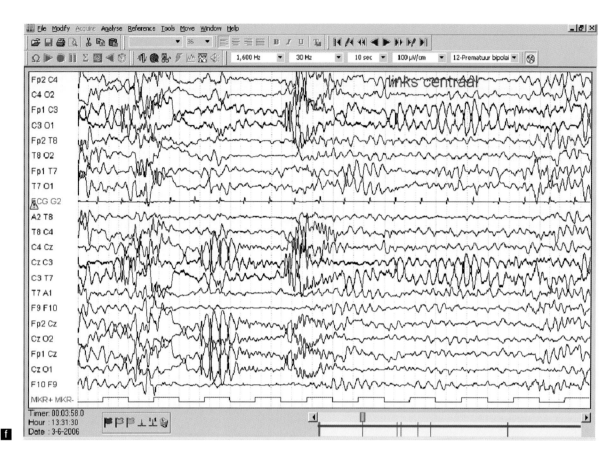

f

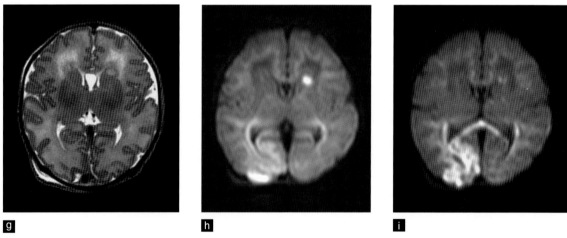

g   h   i

Figure 4.7 *opposite*   A standard EEG was done and multifocal brief ictal discharges were confirmed. Another loading dose of phenobarbitone was given, resulting in control of the seizures, while the EEG background changed to a BS pattern (see also videoclip).

Cranial ultrasound showed some echogenicity in the left thalamus and some periventricular echogenicity. An MRI performed on day 5 showed high signal intensity in the white matter on the T2 spinecho sequence (g) a focal infarction in the left caudate nucleus, as well as in the distribution of the right posterior cerebral artery, best seen on the diffusion weighted imaging (DWI) (h and i). The MR venography showed a possible partial occlusion of the superior sagittal sinus (not shown).

This case is of interest for several reasons. It clearly shows the additional value of the original EEG for distinguishing aEEG changes due to care and seizures, and for identifying subclinical status epilepticus. It also shows that one should continue the aEEG recording when the background pattern has not yet normalized as ictal discharges and even a status epilepticus can occur late during a phase of (probable) secondary energy failure.

Prolonged seizures mimicking continuous normal voltage activity

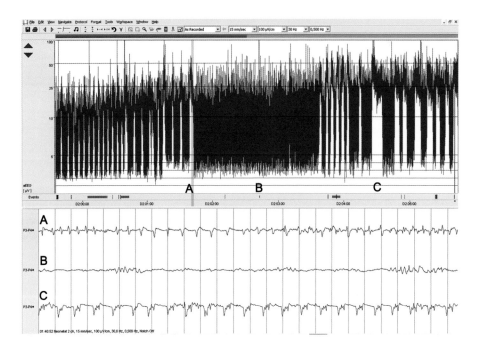

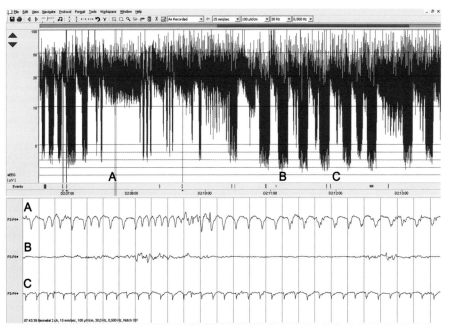

Figure 4.8 This infant was born at 38 gestational weeks with a birthweight of 3055 g. She was initially doing well but developed transient hypoglycemia at 9 h of age (blood glucose 1.2 mmol/l). At 12 h clinical seizures were noted. The two aEEG panels both have a duration of 6 h and were recorded between the first and second day of life. The upper panel (a) shows from the beginning almost 2 h of status epilepticus; a representative sample of the EEG can be seen below at A. Morphine was administered soon after A and resulted in a discontinuous background for 2 h (B). Seizures of different duration recurred; at C the seizure had a duration of more than 10 min. The intensity of the seizure pattern in the second panel (b) can easily be misinterpreted at first glance. Prolonged seizures raised the aEEG pattern (A), where almost 3 h of continuously ongoing seizures were recorded (trace has been slightly pruned), while the relatively brief, but broader part of the trace represents the only part where no seizures were detected (B). At C there are, again, prolonged seizures of duration greater than 10 min. The seizures were difficult to control in spite of treatment with phenobarbitone, midazolam, lidocaine, fos-fenytoin, and pentobarbital.

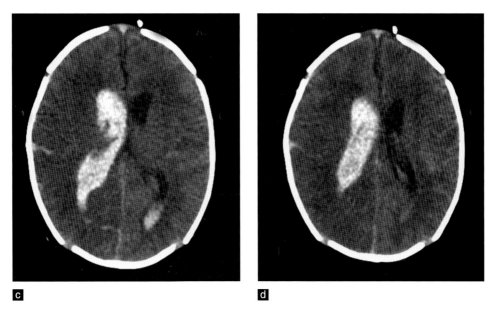

c   d

Figure 4.8 *opposite and above*   Cranial ultrasound and CT scan (c, d) showed a predominantly right-sided intraventricular hemorrhage and decreased attenuation of the adjacent white matter, for which she later required a ventriculoperitoneal shunt.

'Uncoupling', i.e. electroclinical seizures continue as subclinical seizures

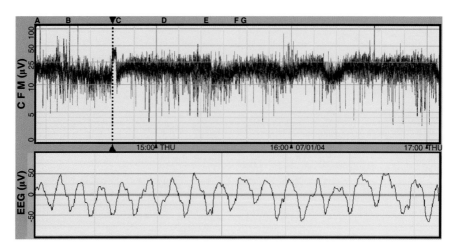

C, drop in saturation; D, lidocaine loading dose; E, inserting umbilical lines.

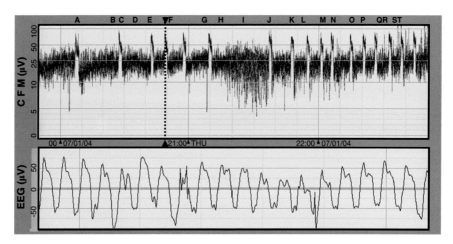

A, drip placement; B, abdominal X-ray; C–F, saturation drop; G, increased blood pressure, smacking; H, midazolam loading dose; I, midazolam continuous infusion; J, increased blood pressure; K–P, seizure, Q, insertion central line; R and S, midazolam increased; T, seizure.

Figure 4.9 *opposite and above* This male infant was born at 41 weeks' gestation with a birthweight of 4055 g. During delivery there was meconium-stained amniotic fluid. His Apgar scores were 8 and 9 at 1 and 5 min, respectively, and he initially went to the postnatal ward. However, when he was almost 1 day old he developed suspected seizures with pallor and tonic eye deviation. He was admitted to the neonatal unit and given a loading dose of phenobarbitone (20 mg/kg iv). He was then referred to the regional level III NICU for evaluation. He needed support with mechanical ventilation due to respiratory failure after administration of several antiepileptic drugs. Phenobarbitone was continued for 3 months following discharge, in view of the long status epilepticus and a family history of epilepsy. He survived and his development is within the normal range at 30 months of age (DQ 96 with the Griffiths developmental scale).

aEEG was started when he was almost 24 h old (panel 1, a). Overall background activity was continuous and of normal voltage, with some variability. A transient elevation of the aEEG trace was seen around 30 min after the recording was started. The original EEG below confirmed the epileptic nature, showing 2 Hz rhythmic spike-wave complexes (see also videoclip). Lidocaine was given shortly afterwards (D); it did not change the electrocortical background pattern, and no more seizures were detected in this trace. The second panel (b) shows 17 seizures in the 3-h aEEG trace. Several annotations, including clinical symptoms and administration of drugs, are made and facilitate the interpretation of the recording. Midazolam was started at H, and results in a transient depression of the background activity before the next seizure arises after about 25 min.

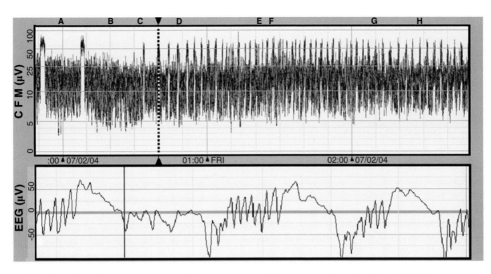

A, loading dose clonazepam; B and C, care; D and E, increased midazolam; H, clonazepom increased.

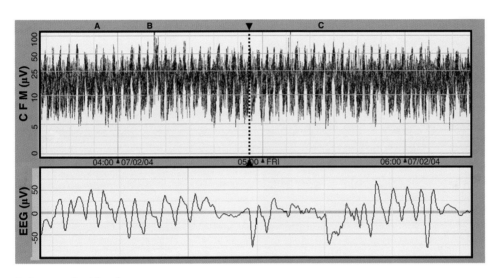

A, increased midazolam.

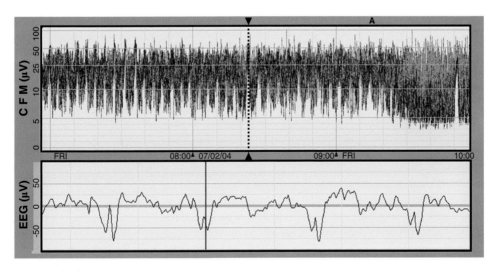

A, phenobarbitone.

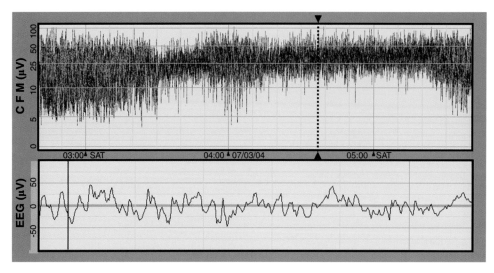

f

32h.

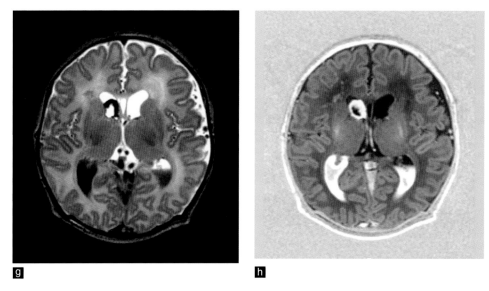

g

h

Figure 4.9 *continued*   In the third panel (c) a subclinical status epilepticus emerged ('saw-tooth pattern' in the aEEG), which was not stopped by increasing the midazolam (H) or by administration of clonazepam (A). The status epilepticus continued in panels (d) and (e), before it was interrupted by another loading dose of phenobarbitone in panel (e) at A. The EEG of panel (e) before the phenobarbitone shows complexes of 2–3 s, consisting of series of polyspikes followed by a large slow wave. The last panel (f), taken one day later at 32 h after birth, shows a normal voltage pattern with the onset of sleep–wake cycling. The background pattern in this infant remained normal or slightly discontinuous almost throughout the RS and SE period and only became briefly discontinuous when the status epilepticus was interrupted with phenobarbitone.

Cranial ultrasound on admission showed a bilateral intraventricular hemorrhage with mild right-sided parenchymal involvement as well. This was later confirmed by MRI, performed on day 6 (T2 weighted spinecho sequence (g) and inversion recovery sequence (h) are shown).

This case illustrates how valuable an aEEG recording with a long duration can be. While the seizures were all clinical to start with, the status epilepticus which lasted for 9 h was entirely subclinical. The use of careful marking of all events is well shown in the second panel. Standard EEGs were performed on several occasions to verify the aEEG findings. In spite of the status epilepticus, the electrocortical background was preserved, and the outcome was good at 30 months without recurrence of seizures.

Benign familial neonatal seizures

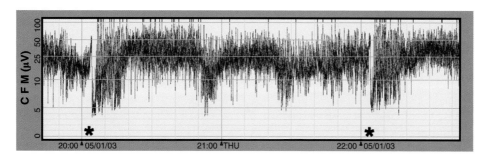

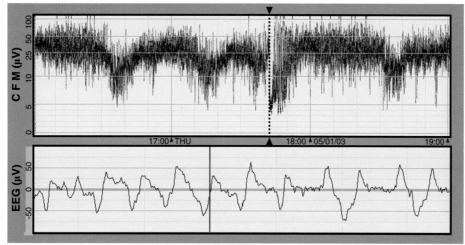

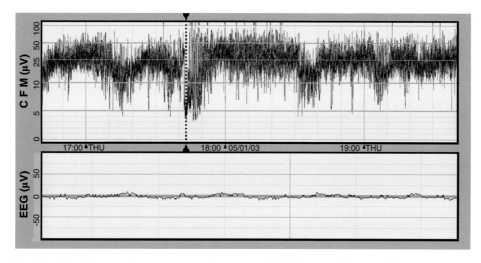

Figure 4.10   This female infant was born at term after a normal delivery with normal Apgar scores. However, repeated clinical seizures were seen within the first 12 h, presenting as abnormal eye movements, staring, tonic stretching of the upper limbs, and cyanosis. The infant was doing well in between the seizures. The mother had a history of seizures during the first 3 months after birth, and a diagnosis of familial benign neonatal seizures was later confirmed in this infant, with a mutation of the KCNQ2 gene which was also present in the mother. Her neurodevelopmental outcome showed a global delay at 3 years of age.

The aEEG shows two ictal discharges in (a) (*) and one in (b). The seizures are recognized as sudden increases in the lower and upper margins, followed by a short period of postictal depression. The original EEG in (b) shows ictal slow-wave activity at about 1 Hz, while the EEG in (c) shows postictal depression. Postictal depression of electrocortical activity is not uncommon, and is more easily seen in less time-compressed aEEG recordings.

5

Hypoxia–ischemia

aEEG AND PERINATAL ASPHYXIA

The neonatal EEG is depressed during and immediately after an acute hypoxic–ischemic insult.[15,102,103] The degree and duration of the EEG depression correlates with the severity of the brain injury.[104,105] During the recovery, the EEG subsequently contains information on the severity of the previous hypoxic–ischemic insult. In newborn infants, the electrocortical activity is a highly sensitive predictor of neurologic outcome when recorded early after a hypoxic–ischemic insult.[12,14,106–108] Several studies have shown that outcome can be accurately predicted from an aEEG during the first hours after birth (see Table 5.1).[42,109–115] These findings were also confirmed by a meta-analysis evaluating aEEG for prediction of outcome.[116] From the eight eligible studies included, there was an overall sensitivity of 91% (95% confidence interval (CI) 87–95%) and a negative likelihood ratio of 0.09 (95% CI 0.06–0.15) for aEEG tracings to accurately predict poor outcome.[42,105,109–113,115] The authors concluded that 'the meta-analysis clearly shows that aEEG is useful in predicting long-term neurodevelopmental outcome in the population of high-risk term infants'. The authors of the meta-analysis also recommended that aEEG should be part of the initial evaluation in full-term infants with suspected hypoxic–ischemic encephalopathy (HIE).

In asphyxiated full-term infants, the aEEG can accurately predict outcome in 80% of the infants at 3 h and in 90% of the infants at 6 h postnatally.[109,110,112] Pattern recognition has mainly been used for classification of aEEG background in asphyxiated infants. However, comparable figures for prediction of outcome were obtained by al Naqeeb et al, who used evaluation of the background amplitudes to classify aEEG recordings in newborn infants with neonatal encephalopathy during the first 6 h of life.[42] Later, another study compared aEEG pattern versus amplitude for prediction of outcome and found that pattern recognition was slightly better than amplitude, although the difference was quite small.[117] The early aEEG background in asphyxiated infants correlates with the degree of neurone-specific enolase in the cerebrospinal fluid, and with cerebral glucose metabolism later in the neonatal period.[118,119] Combining neurologic examination with aEEG performed <12 h after birth further increases predictive accuracy from 75 to 85%.[113,120] A negative relationship was recently found between EEG amplitude measures, Sarnat grades, and MRI abnormality scores. This relationship was strongest for the minimum amplitude measures in both hemispheres. A minimum amplitude of <4 μV was useful in predicting severe MRI abnormalities.[121]

The ability of the aEEG to predict neurologic outcome after hypoxic–ischemic events occurring in moderately preterm infants, or later in the neonatal period or infancy, has not been widely studied, although the scarce data indicate that the aEEG background pattern and the recovery rate are also correlated with outcome.[12]

HYPOTHERMIA

The early aEEG background (<6 h after delivery) has also been used for evaluation of the severity of the hypoxic–ischemic insult in full-term infants before inclusion in intervention studies. In the multicenter

Table 5.1 Predictive values of abnormal background patterns (BS, CLV, FT) during the first 3 and 6 h (12) of life, to predict adverse outcomes (death or handicap). Data modified from references 42, 105, 109, 111, 112, 113, and 117

	Sensitivity (%)	Specificity (%)	Positive predictive value (PPV) (%)	Negative predictive value (NPV) (%)
6 h (Hellström-Westas et al[112]) n=47	95	89	86	96
6 h (Eken et al[111]) n=34	94	79	84	92
6 h (Toet et al[109]) n=68	91	86	86	96
3 h (Toet et al[108]) n=68	85	77	78	84
6 h (al Naqeeb et al[42]) n=56	93	70	77	90
12 h (Shalak et al[113]) n=15	79	89	73	91
6 h (vanRooij et al[105]) n=161	83	85	88	91
6 h (Shany et al[117]) n=39	100	87	69	100

hypothermia study, no effect of hypothermia was noted on outcome in those with the most severe baseline aEEG changes (n=46), with severe suppression of background activity and seizures (odds ratio 1.8; 95% CI 0.49–6.4, p=0.51). By contrast, in the remaining 172 infants outcome was more favorable in cooled infants than in controls (odds ratio 0.47; 95% CI 0.26–0.87, p=0.021). The number needed to treat was six (95% CI 3–27).[43]

Moderate hypothermia is now increasingly used for clinical intervention after perinatal asphyxia. It is likely that the old figures for prediction of outcome from aEEG will be changed when estimated in relation to this new intervention. Nevertheless, the aEEG prior to cooling will still indicate infants with the highest risks. Possible effects from cooling on aEEG amplitudes were evaluated by Horan et al, who calculated minimum and maximum amplitudes from aEEGs of 26 infants during extracorporeal membrane oxygenation (ECMO) treatment.[122] Six of the infants served as controls and were not cooled, the 20 other children were cooled to different body temperatures (34 to 36°C) for different time periods (24 to 48 h). The aEEG amplitude during the 6 h prior to rewarming (from 34 to 36°C) was compared with the aEEG amplitude during 6 h after rewarming, but there was no difference in amplitudes. Although not currently evaluated in the clinical setting, experimental data indicate that hypothermia decreases the amplitude of seizures.[93] Consequently, there is a risk that seizures could become more difficult to identify in the aEEG, if the EEG trace is not considered.

POSTASPHYCTIC SEIZURES

The presence of epileptic seizure activity does not seem to be as strong a predictor as the background activity. Seizures did not seem to affect outcome in asphyxiated infants with mild HIE or a normal EEG. However, seizures were correlated with worse outcome in infants with moderate to severe HIE or a low voltage EEG.[123–125] In a recent study of 56 full-term infants an aEEG diagnosis of status epilepticus (SE) background activity at the onset of SE was noted to be the main predictor of neurodevelopmental outcome. The duration of the SE was only of predictive value in a subgroup of 48 infants with HIE.[126] Furthermore, the postnatal age when postasphyctic seizures develop could be correlated with outcome, although different results have been obtained.[118,120] Onset beyond 12 h of neonatal seizures is more common in neonatal stroke than HIE, and these infants are more likely to present with hemiconvulsions. Table 5.2 presents a summary of predictive features in aEEG, modified from reference 118.

REACTIVITY TO CARE

Reactivity to caregiving is seen as a short transient rise in the aEEG background, when the aEEG is discontinuous and the infant is not too ill or heavily sedated. Reactivity is not usually clearly discernible in infants with a CNV aEEG background and can be confused with an ictal discharge (see Figure 3.2), but with

Table 5.2 Summary of impact of different aEEG features for prediction of outcome in asphyxiated full-term infants (modified from reference 118)

	Age		
	0–12 h	12–24 h	24–48 h
Background pattern	++	+	–
Epileptic seizures	–	+	–
Sleep–wake cycling	+	+	–
Reactivity to care	–	–	–

access to the original EEG a distinction can nowadays be made.

RECOVERY OF aEEG BACKGROUND AFTER 6 POSTNATAL HOURS

The electrocortical background normalizes and becomes CNV in most full-term infants within 1–2 weeks following a severe hypoxic–ischemic insult. In a large study of 160 full-term infants admitted and recorded with aEEG within 6 h after birth, 65 had an initial FT or CLV pattern and 25 an initial BS pattern. The background pattern recovered to CNV within 24 h in 6 of the 65 infants (9%) in the FT/CLV group, and 5 of them were normal at follow-up. In the BS group, the background pattern improved to normal voltage in 12 of the 25 infants (48%) within 24 h. Of these infants, 2 survived with mild disability, and 4 were normal. The patients who did not recover within 24 h either died in the neonatal period or survived with a severe disability. Although the actual number of infants with background recovery within 24 h was small (9%), more than half of these infants (61%) had a normal or mildly abnormal outcome. Continuation of aEEG recording and intensive care treatment in the severely asphyxiated infant for at least 24 h is therefore warranted, as there is a chance of recovery with a good neurodevelopmental outcome.[105]

Burst suppression is usually a marker of severe brain damage in full-term infants and seems to constitute a disconnection in brain circuits between the cerebral cortex and deep layers, e.g. the thalamus.[126–128] In term infants with discontinuous EEG, the IBI is the EEG feature that correlated best with outcome.

A predominant IBI of more than 30s is associated with a 100% probability of severe neurologic disability or death, and an 86% risk for development of epilepsy.[126] Postmortem neuropathologic investigations have shown a direct relationship between the number of damaged neurons and the EEG background activity in both full-term and preterm infants.[129,130] Aso and colleagues found that EEG inactivity was correlated with widespread encephalomalacia engaging the cerebral cortex, corpus striatum, thalamus, midbrain, and pons in postmortem studies of newborn infants.[129] Burst suppression was also related to multifocal severe brain damage, but no damage to any specific brain structures was identified in these infants.[129] In asphyxiated piglets the burst recovery (occurrence and duration) was also predictive of outcome.[131]

SLEEP–WAKE CYCLING

Another important feature is the development of sleep–wake cycling during the recovery phase following a hypoxic–ischemic insult. Although sleep–wake cycling is noted to develop eventually in almost all children who survive (95%), and even in 8% of those who do not survive the neonatal period, the time of onset is associated with the severity of HIE, being 7, 33, and 62 h for Sarnat grade I, II, and III, respectively (see Figure 5.1).[132] Newborns with seizure discharges developed sleep–wake cycling with a delay of 30.5 h. Good outcome was associated with earlier onset of sleep–wake cycling and normal pattern. The difference in the median Griffiths' DQs in newborns who started sleep–wake cycling before/after 36 h was 8.5 points. The good/poor neurodevelopmental outcome was predicted correctly by the onset of sleep–wake cycling before/after 36 h in 82% of newborns. A significant delay of the onset was seen only when more than two antiepileptic drugs were administered.

HYPOXIC–ISCHEMIC BRAIN INJURY DUE TO CAUSES OTHER THAN PERINATAL ASPHYXIA

Critically ill and unstable neonates may experience several events during intensive care that may negatively affect brain function, e.g. periods with low or unstable oxygenation and blood pressure. Such high-risk infants include babies with congenital heart defects and congenital diaphragmatic hernias, infants with persistent pulmonary hypertension of the newborn, infants developing pneumothoraces, and infants with severe infections. With the aEEG it is possible to follow the impact on the brain in such infants. By combining regional cerebral oxygen saturation (rSO_2), fractional cerebral tissue oxygen extraction (FTOE) measured by near-infrared spectroscopy (NIRS), and aEEG after perinatal asphyxia, it was shown that rSO_2 increased and FTOE decreased in the infants with an adverse outcome, but these alterations were only significantly different after the first 24 h. aEEG, however, showed the closest and also the earliest relationship with outcome, within hours after birth.[133]

The EEG background in infants needing ECMO seems to be predictive of neurologic outcome, and subclinical seizure activity during ECMO treatment is not uncommon.[134–136] There was no acute change in aEEG background during ECMO, nor were there lateralizing effects in a small group of neonates ($n = 20$). An abnormal aEEG predicted death or moderate to severe intracranial neuropathology (moderate to severe hydrocephaly, ischemia, infarction, or hemorrhage documented on neuroimaging or autopsy) with sensitivity = 1.0, specificity = 0.75, positive predictive value = 0.86, and negative predictive value = 1.0.

SUMMARY

- In full-term asphyxiated infants, a CNV background, or a continuous but slightly periodic background pattern with normal amplitude within the first hours of life, is predictive of good outcome.

- In full-term asphyxiated infants, abnormal aEEG patterns, including discontinuous patterns such as BS and electrocerebral inactivity (i.e. flat), or extremely low-voltage patterns, are predictive of poor outcome (death or severe handicap).

- Most asphyxiated infants with an early BS aEEG background have a poor neurologic outcome. However, some infants with rapid recovery of the aEEG (during the first 24 h) survive without handicap.

- In order to assess recovery of the background activity and time for onset of sleep–wake cycling, aEEG recordings should be continued for a minimum of 48–72 h.

- Sedative and anticonvulsive medications can affect the aEEG background activity and contribute to a more uncertain evaluation of the aEEG pattern.

- At least one standard EEG should always be recorded early during the neonatal course. Furthermore, after the first few days the standard EEG is superior for evaluation of detailed electrocortical abnormalities since the expected findings are subtler and sometimes not possible to detect with aEEG.

Time at onset of sleep-wake cycling and outcome after birth asphyxia

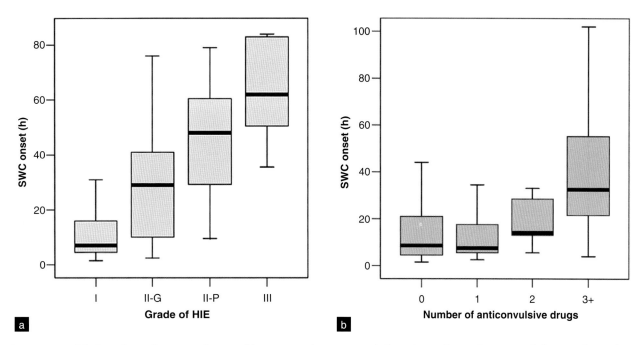

Figure 5.1 (a) Correlation between degree of hypoxic–ischemic encephalopathy and time for onset of sleep–wake cycling in hours after birth. Grade II-G denotes infants with HIE II and good outcome, while II-P denotes infants with HIE II and poor outcome.

(b) The number of anticonvulsive drugs in asphyxiated infants in relation to time at onset of sleep–wake cycling. From reference 132 with permission.

Mild HIE with good outcome

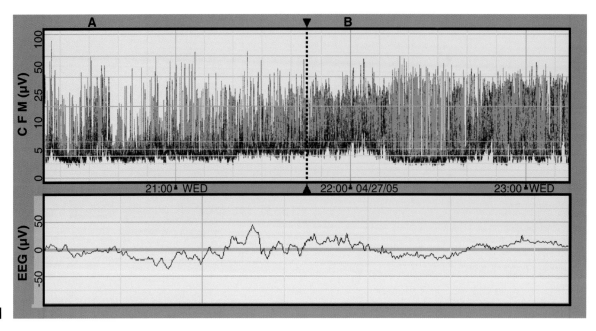

Age 5½ h; A, care; B, phenobarbitone.

Figure 5.2 This female infant was born at 41 weeks' gestation by an emergency Cesarean section because of fetal heart rate changes. Her birthweight was 3825 g. Her Apgar scores were 2, 3, and 3, the umbilical artery pH was 6.70 with a base excess of –28 mmol/l, and arterial lactate was 14 mmol/l. The first hemoglobin was only 7.3 mmol/l, suggesting a feto–maternal transfusion, which was subsequently confirmed. Outcome at 19 months was just within the normal range with a developmental quotient (DQ) on the Griffiths developmental scale of 94, although with a delay in speech development.

Cranial ultrasound showed mildly increased echogenicity in the thalami. No MRI was performed as she showed such a rapid recovery.

aEEG was started soon after admission and showed a BS pattern at 5.5 h, with increasing amplitude and burst density during the following hours, except for the hour following administration of phenobarbitone, at B in panel a, which resulted in a transient decrease of burst density. The phenobarbitone was given since seizures were suspected clinically, but they were not confirmed on the aEEG or single-channel EEG. The corresponding EEG trace below the aEEG indicates a slightly discontinuous background, although some very slow drifts of the baseline and non-specific rapid low-voltage activity make the interpretation difficult. In panel b, a rapid recovery of the background occurs which changes from discontinuous to continuous when she is around 9 h old. There is a slight discrepancy between the aEEG, which looks discontinuous, and the corresponding 7 s of EEG below, which look continuous. A running display of the EEG would show that the background was still discontinuous but that continuous periods of increasing duration appeared. Panel c, starting at 31 h, shows a continuous normal voltage pattern with sleep–wake cycling.

This severely asphyxiated infant with feto–maternal transfusion initially showed a markedly abnormal background pattern, at 6 h of age, with rapid normalization to a CNV pattern within 12 h of age, and emerging sleep–wake cycling before 36 h after birth. Around 50% of asphyxiated infants who display recovery of an initial BS pattern to CNV before 24 h have a good outcome.

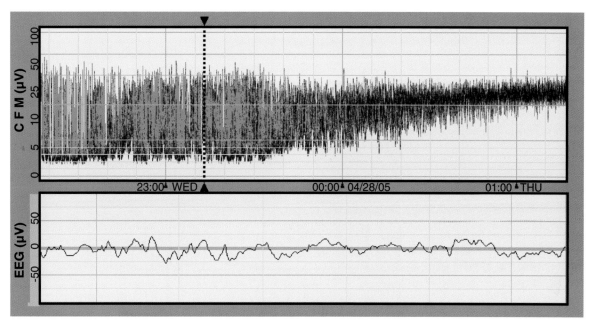

Age 8 h.

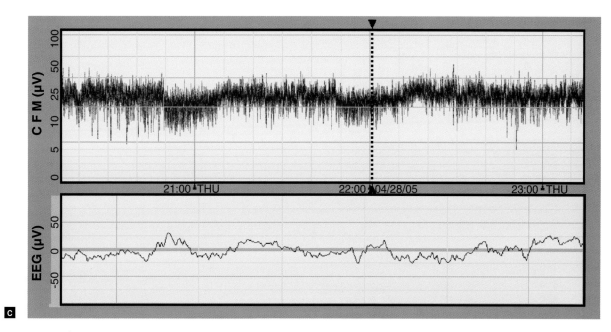

Age 31 h.

Rapid recovery of abnormal background pattern

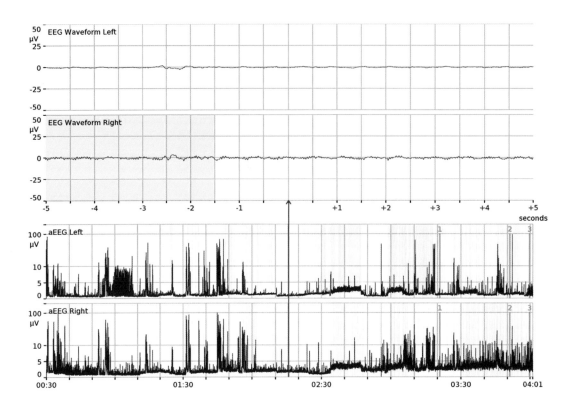

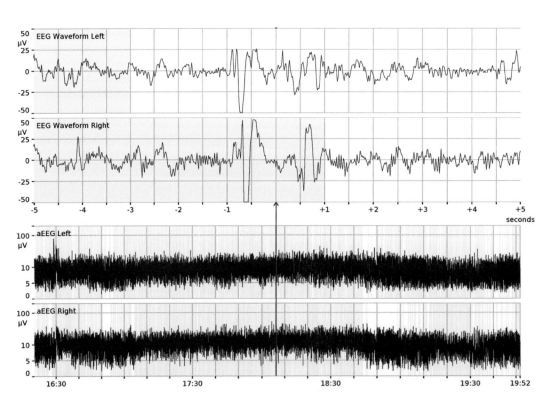

Figure 5.3 *opposite*   This male infant was born at 40 weeks' gestation and had a birthweight of 3580 g. He was born by ventouse extraction because of fetal bradycardia and meconium-stained liquor. His Apgar scores were 3, 4, and 8, at 1, 5, and 10 minutes, respectively. His umbilical arterial pH was 6.81, with a base excess of –23.6 mmol/l. He was intubated and ventilated and recovered until there was a second episode of asphyxia, when he required cardiac massage and intravenous epinephrine. This deterioration was due to a tension pneumothorax, which was not immediately recognized. Once the pneumothorax was drained he recovered. Following these two episodes of hypoxia–ischemia he was transferred to the NICU. His first arterial lactate at 6 h of age was only 4.8 mmol/l. He was given a loading dose of phenobarbitone in the local hospital but subsequently did not develop any clinical or subclinical seizures. He made a rapid recovery and his outcome at 18 months of age was well within the normal range, with a DQ of 110.

Cranial ultrasound showed a mild increase in echogenicity in the thalami and his MRI performed on day 5 only showed a small amount of fresh blood in the posterior fossa and a small subdural hemorrhage without any evidence of ischemic changes on diffusion weighted imaging (DWI).

The aEEG, which was started immediately after admission at 5.5 h of age, was almost completely inactive during the first 3 h of recording, then the beginning of a low-amplitude BS pattern can be seen (a). Within 12 h, however, there was recovery to a more continuous background pattern, already showing some early sleep–wake cycling within 24 h after birth, when the recording in panel b begins. Monitoring was continued for 48 h, but no seizures were ever seen. A standard EEG was performed at 24 h of age and showed a mildly discontinuous pattern with a *tracé alternans*, but also more discontinuous periods with isolated sharp waves in the central and temporal region bilaterally.

This very unusual case shows that even in the presence of an inactive recording, recovery may be seen and may even be associated with a good outcome if the electrocortical background normalizes within the first 24 h which is also shown in reference 105.

Postasphyxia intervention with moderate hypothermia

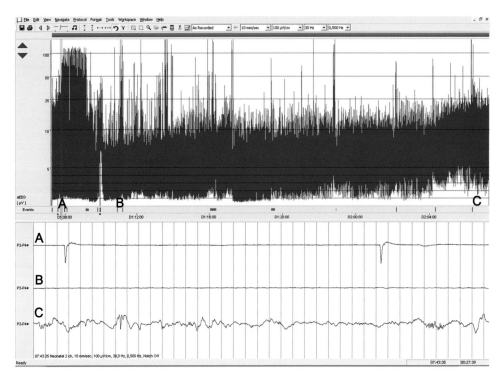

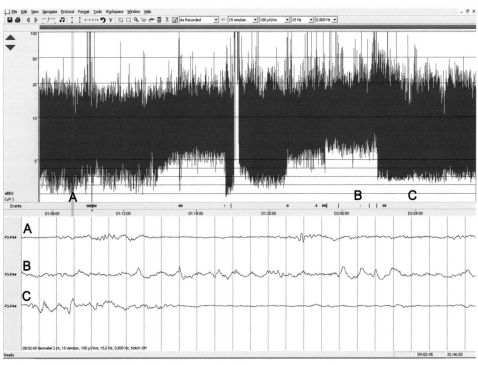

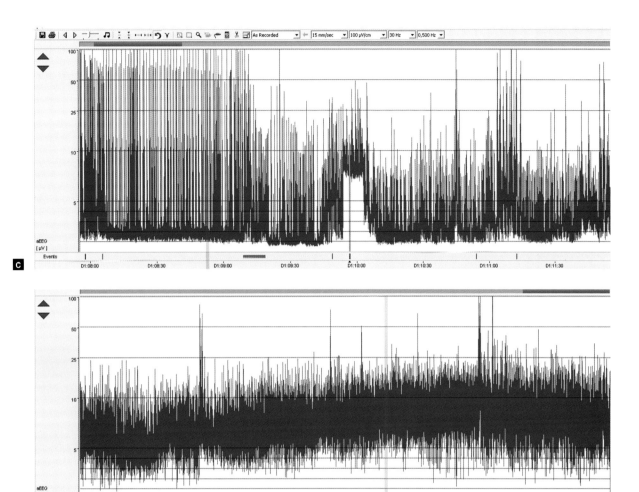

Figure 5.4 *opposite and above* **Case 1** (a–d) This full-term infant was delivered in an ambulance, and needed resuscitation following delivery. The infant showed intermittent gasping but was otherwise unresponsive at arrival to the hospital 20 min later. The two upper panels (a,b) show very compressed aEEG trends, each of 23–24 hours' duration. Panel (a) shows the aEEG during the first 24 h of life. One hour after arrival there was no EEG activity, only gasping, which could be misinterpreted since it looks like a BS pattern in the aEEG. However, it was obvious when looking at the infant and the simultaneous EEG that it was the gasping that caused the monorhythmic brief waves of activity (panel a, A). The infant was included in the TOBY (total body cooling) trial after parental consent and was randomized to cooling, which started at B. The electrocortical background recovers gradually during the following hours and is mainly continuous at C, when the infant was 24 h old. A nurse also made a note here 'seems to be more awake now'. Panel (b) shows a gradual recovery during the following 24 h, although some periods are still discontinuous (A). The interruption of the aEEG trace is due to a loose electrode. Midazolam was given between B and C for a suspected clinical seizure, which was not verified by the aEEG. Panels (c) and (d) contain two 4-h displays of the aEEG, as they are more commonly seen, from the beginning and the end of panel (a). The raised aEEG trace in the upper trace is due to recording of a full standard EEG. This infant has normal neurodevelopmental outcome at 15 months.

Postasphyxia intervention with moderate hypothermia

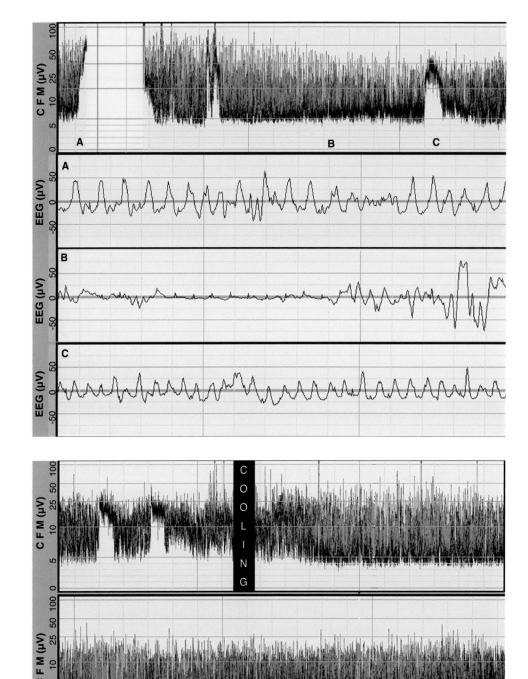

Figure 5.4 *continued*

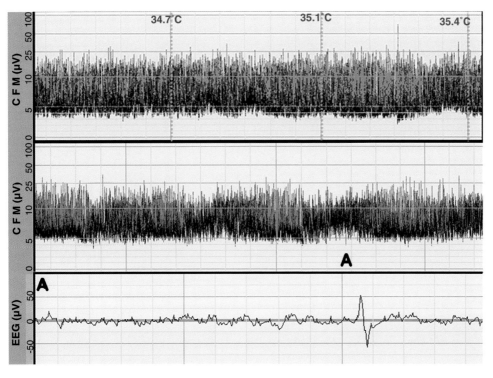

g

Figure 5.4 *opposite and above* **Case 2** (e–g) This boy was born at 42 weeks' gestation following spontaneous labor with rupture of membranes on the day of delivery. Meconium-stained amniotic fluid and fetal decelerations with poor variability on the CTG led to an emergency Cesarean section. Apgar scores were 3, 5, and 9 at 1, 5, and 10 min, respectively. At 30 min he became apneic and seizures were questioned.

The aEEG started at 3 h 45 min of age, with corresponding EEG traces below. By (A) he had an episode of clinical and electrical seizures. Lines were inserted and the aEEG was accidentally disconnected. A loading dose of phenobarbitone (20 mg/kg iv) was given. The aEEG background showed a low-amplitude BS pattern with ECG artifacts clearly visible during the interburst intervals (B). There were no further clinical seizures, although subclinical seizures emerged later (C).

The upper aEEG in panel (f) begins 5 h after birth, and shows two seizures in the beginning of the trace. Hypothermia was commenced as selective head cooling and mild hypothermia (rectal temperature 34–34.5°C). A second dose of phenobarbitone (20 mg/kg iv) was given during this recording and clonazepam (100 µg/kg) was added later.

The lower aEEG in panel (f) shows the aEEG before and after the start of rewarming 72 hours later at (A); the corresponding EEG is taken before rewarming. The infant was treated with mechanical ventilation and received a continuous infusion of morphine, 10 µg/kg/h. The upper aEEG panel g shows the aEEG during rewarming; the figures above the aEEG show the rectal temperature.

The lower aEEG with corresponding EEG in panel (g) shows the end of the 8 h of rewarming (A). The rectal temperature here was 36.0°C. The aEEG is more continuous and shows imminent sleep–wake cycling, and the EEG voltage is slightly higher than before rewarming.

The baby was abnormal neurologically for the first week, stiff and slow to feed; home and breast/bottle fed by 16 days. The MRI at 9 days of age was reported to be normal. Clinical examination by 3 months was normal apart from hearing loss. *Case contributed by Marianne Thoresen and Xun Liu.*

Moderate HIE with signs of secondary energy failure

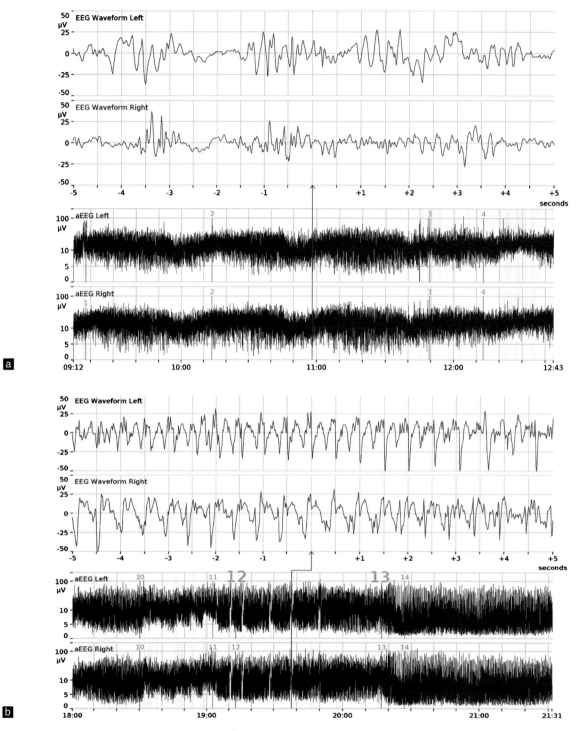

Marker 12: drop in saturation; Marker 13: start midazolam.

Figure 5.5 This male infant was born at 40 weeks' gestation with a birthweight of 3160 g. He was delivered by Cesarean section due to lack of progress of the dilation and a microblood analysis showing a pH of 7.18. His Apgar scores were 8, 9, and 9 at 1, 5, and 10 minutes, respectively. The umbilical artery pH was said to be 7.31. He was admitted with his mother to the postnatal ward, where he was noted to develop seizures when he was 14 h old. A loading dose of phenobarbitone (20 mg/kg iv) was given at 23 h and he was referred to the regional NICU. He was discharged home at 2 weeks and had a good outcome with DQ of 115 at 36 months (Griffiths developmental assessment scale).

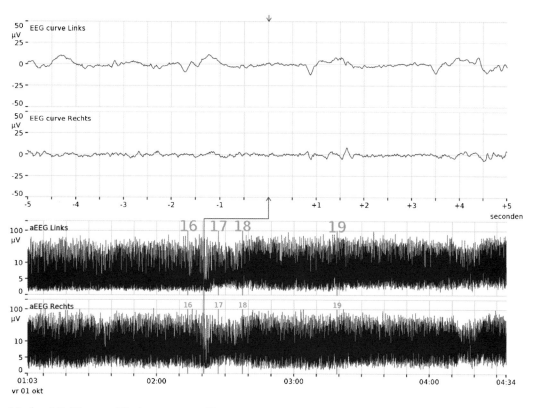

Marker 16–17: care; 18: desaturation; 19: care.

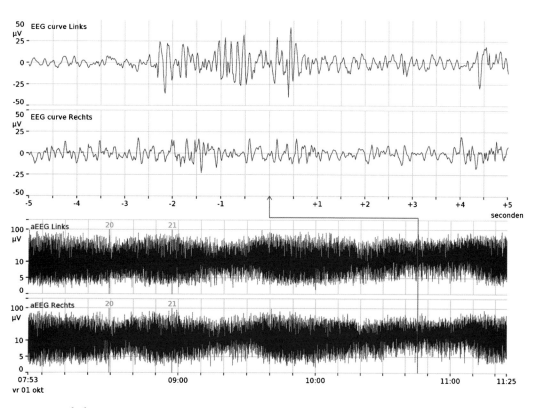

Figure 5.5 *opposite and above*

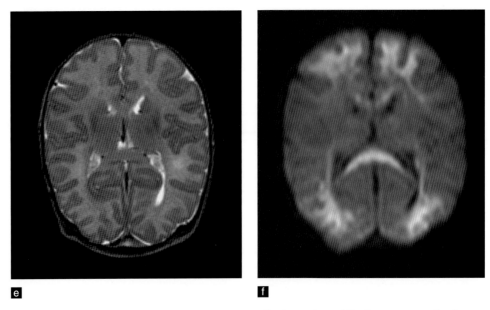

Figure 5.5 *continued*   The aEEG started 26 h after delivery, initially showed a mildly discontinuous background pattern with some variation, but not a normal sleep-wake cycling pattern (a). Twelve hours later a more discontinuous pattern was seen with very short elevations of the trace (b). These were confirmed to be ictal discharges on the original EEG (spike-wave activity of about 4 Hz on the left and 2 Hz on the right). A drop in saturation was seen at marker 12 and midazolam was given at marker 13 in panel b. In panel c a downward deflection of the tracing is noted, which correlates with spike-wave activity in the left EEG tracing. In panel d, at 36 h of age, an emerging sleep–wake cycling pattern can be seen.

His cranial ultrasound scan on arrival showed increased periventricular echogenicity. A diagnosis of bilateral watershed infarcts was made with MRI, performed on day 4, and the changes were especially well appreciated using DWI. Both T2 spinecho sequence (e) and DWI (f) are shown. (Figure 5.5(f) reproduced with permission from Groenendaal F, de Vries LS. Images in neonatal medicine: watershed infarcts in the fullterm neonatal brain. Arch Dis Child Fetal Neonatal Ed 2005; 90: F488.)

This example shows that registration should be performed for at least 48 h following the perinatal problems, even when a good background pattern is seen to start with.

Severe HIE with secondary energy failure and other complications

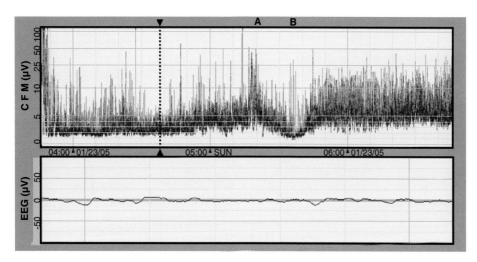

Registration started 3½ h after birth. A, care; B, severe hypotension.

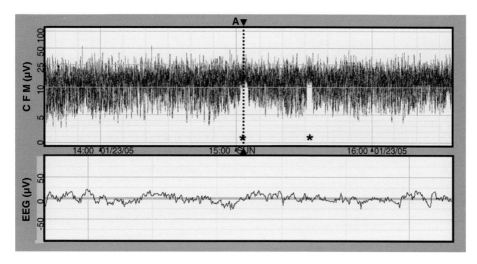

Age 13 h after birth. A, care.

Figure 5.6 This male infant was born at 40 weeks' gestation and had a birthweight of 3800 g. He was born by emergency Cesarean section due to placental abruption. His Apgar scores were 2, 4, and 6 at 1, 5, and 10 minutes, respectively. The umbilical artery pH was 6.77. He was intubated and ventilated after delivery but collapsed again one hour later, due to severe anemia (Hb 6.8 mmol/l) and hypotension, and required resuscitation and iv epinephrine. He was transfused and the Hb on arrival in the regional NICU was 7.4 mmol/l, and the arterial lactate was 27 mmol/l. He continued to be critically ill and needed full inotropic support, and high-frequency ventilation with inhaled nitric oxide (NO). He was also diagnosed with antenatal bowel perforation and required surgery on the first day. In spite of all support, he showed multiorgan failure and severe brain injury and died on day 2.

aEEG was started at 3.5 h of age, and showed initially a severely depressed background pattern continuous low voltage (CLV), with gradual recovery and again transient deterioration during a severely hypotensive period (a). The electrocortical background at 13 h had improved remarkably to a continuous voltage pattern, which is seen also in the single-channel EEG below the aEEG in the second panel (b). Two periods of suspected seizures in the aEEG (marked *) were not confirmed by the original EEG, and at least during the first period (A) care was given. At about 24 h of age (c), prolonged as well as shorter ictal discharges developed during surgery. Some of these discharges were initially suspected to be artifacts due to electrical interference. However, after adjusting the scale of the EEG (check the difference between the first two panels and the other traces), it could be confirmed that the high-voltage activity in the aEEG was due to the high-voltage epileptic discharges in the original EEG (panels c–e). Clear spike-wave activity can be seen in the original EEG in panels c and d and polyspike-wave activity in panel e.

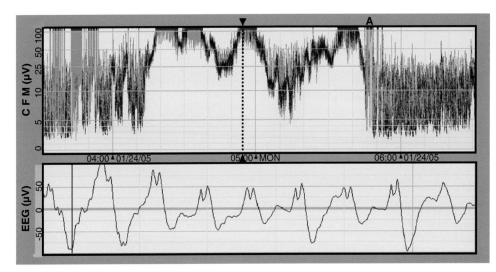

Age 26 h after birth. A, end surgery.

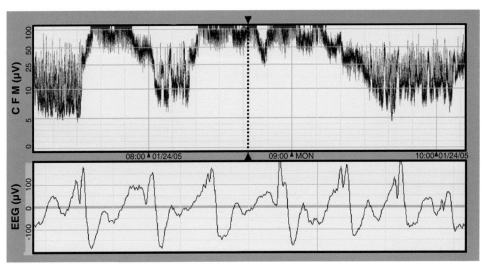

Age 29 h after birth.

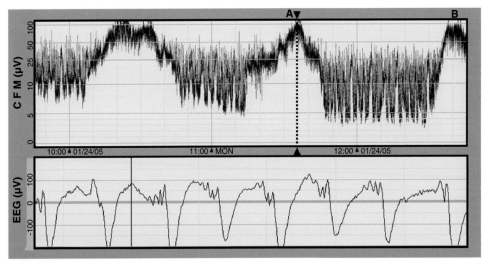

Age 33 h after birth. A, care; B, lidocaine loading dose.

Figure 5.6 *continued* This example shows the importance of continuing the recording for at least 48 h after birth in complicated cases, even when an initial good recovery is seen. Although probably not the case in this infant who was critically ill for a prolonged time, ictal discharges can develop after the first 24 h during a period of secondary energy failure in severely asphyxiated infants. The original EEG in this case revealed the epileptic nature of the suspected artifacts in the aEEG.

Moderate HIE with fair outcome

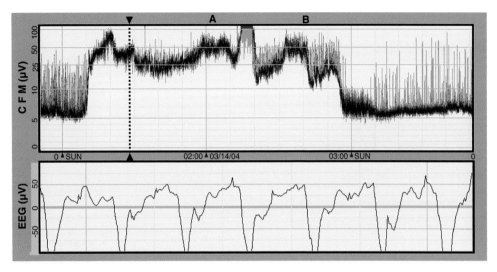

Age 12 h. A, Lidocaine; B, midazolam.

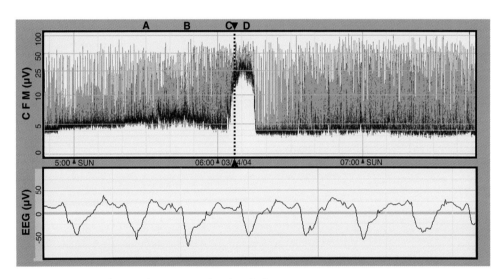

A and B, care; C, lipsmacking; D, midazolam bolus.

Figure 5.7 This female infant was born at term with a birthweight of 4220 g. The pregnancy was complicated by pregnancy-induced diabetes, and decreased fetal movements one day prior to delivery. An emergency Cesarean section was performed due to fetal heart rate changes; there was meconium-stained amniotic fluid. Her Apgar scores were 2, 8, and 9 at 1, 5, and 10 minutes, respectively. The umbilical artery pH was 6.82, the base excess −23 mmol/l, and the arterial lactate 22 mmol/l. She was initially admitted to the high-care unit of a local hospital. She had several low blood glucose levels (0.7, 1.8, and 0.9 mmol/l) and developed her first clinical seizure at 10 h of age. She was given a loading dose (20 mg/kg) of phenobarbitone. She was then intubated and transferred to the regional NICU. She needed ventilation and NO inhalation because of severe persistent pulmonary hypertension of the newborn (PPHN) and was given high doses of dopamine, dobutamine, and hydrocortisone to sustain the blood pressure. She was last seen when 3 years old. She developed a mild diplegia and had a developmental score of 86 on the Griffiths developmental assessment scale.

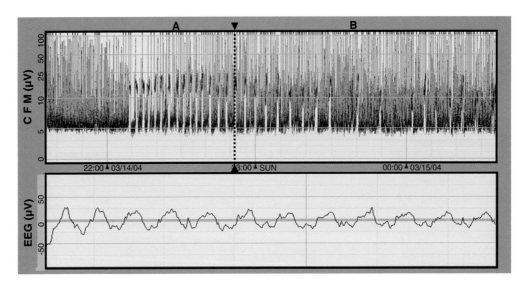

Age 36 h. A and B, midazolam bolus.

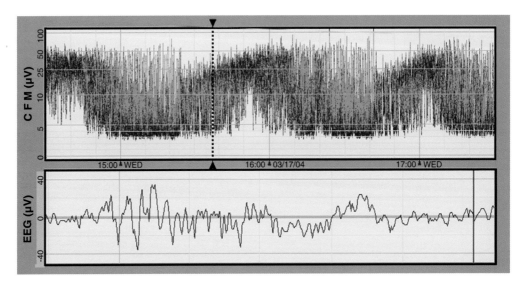

Day 5.

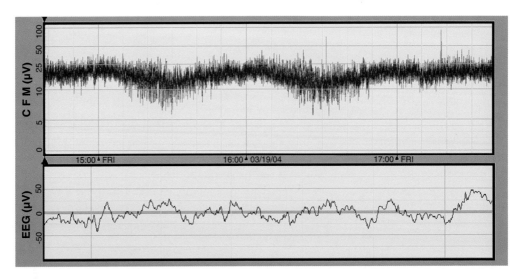

Day 7.

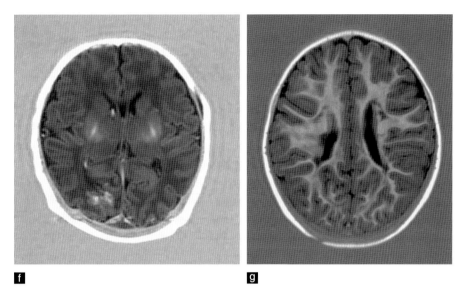

Figure 5.7 *opposite and above*   The aEEG was started immediately after admission, 12 hours after birth (a). The initial aEEG background shows a depressed BS pattern for 20 min. During insertion of the umbilical lines a sustained rise of the trace was noted, which was initially considered to be due to manipulation of the infant. Once the lines were in and the recording was reviewed, it became obvious that this was a very prolonged subclinical status epilepticus, with slow sharp and slow wave complexes with a duration of about 1.5 s. Lidocaine was initially administered but was unable to stop the seizures. Midazolam was then given and the status was stopped after 1.5 h; a reversal to a depressed (low amplitude, sparse burst pattern) BS pattern was seen. Three hours later another ictal discharge was seen, with a duration of 10 min on a 'sparse' BS background, and another loading dose of midazolam was given (b). At 36 h she had another episode of status epilepticus, with a decrease in ictal discharges after administration of midazolam (c). Also note that the lower margin of the trace is above 5 µV throughout the recording in the panels a–c, shown, probably since the EEG is so depressed that other, extracranial, activity is picked up in the recording. Panels d and e show recovery with emerging sleep–wake cycling at the end of the first week, on day 5 still with very discontinuous periods, but on day 7 the aEEG looks normal.

Her cranial ultrasound showed some increase in periventricular echogenicity. An MRI was performed on day 4 and showed an area of hemorrhagic infarction in the right occipital lobe (inversion recovery sequence) and more scattered lesions in the periventricular white matter (f). The inversion recovery sequence at 2 years of age showed more diffuse white matter loss and areas of gliosis within the white matter and mild ventriculomegaly (g).

When a sustained rise in the aEEG is seen, even though external interference on the aEEG can be suspected, the original EEG has to be examined for suspected seizure activity. This case also shows the utility of long-term (here 7 days) monitoring. The early depressed background, the status epilepticus, and the late onset of sleep–wake cycling were all indicative of an increased risk for neurologic handicap.

Severe HIE and poor outcome

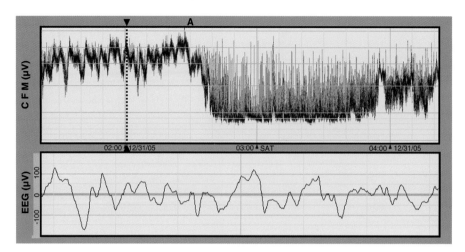

Age 6 h. A, phenobarbitone loading dose.

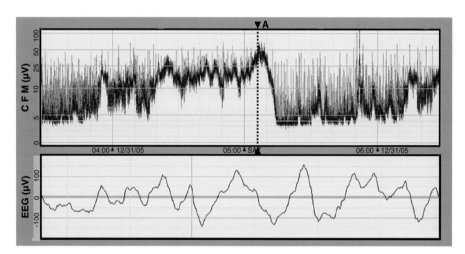

A, midazolam bolus.

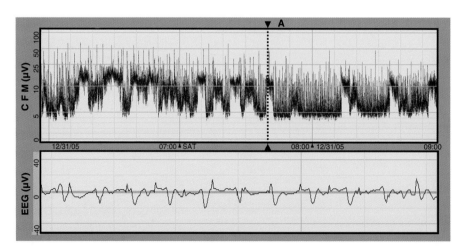

A, lidocaine bolus.

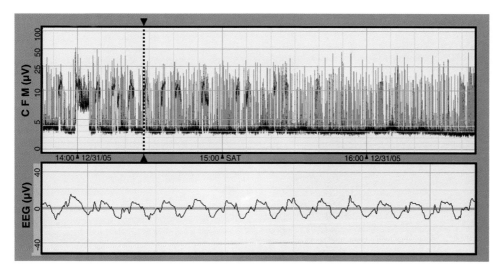

Age 21 h.

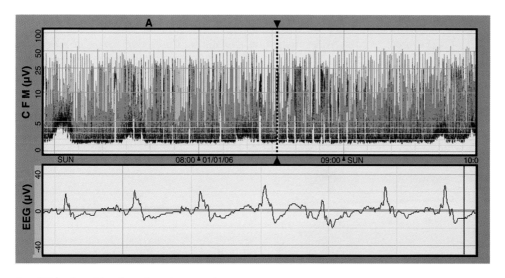

Age 36 h. A, midazolam dose increased.

Figure 5.8 *opposite and above*   This female infant was born at 40 weeks and had a birthweight of 3290 g. She was delivered by emergency Cesarean section, due to fetal heart rate changes, but the mother had noticed decreased fetal movements already one day prior to delivery. Apgar scores were 0, 7, and 9 at 1, 5, and 10 minutes, respectively. The umbilical artery pH was 6.77 with a base excess of –26 mmol/l. She was resuscitated after delivery, including cardiac massage and administration of epinephrine. The first blood glucose was 0.9 mmol/l, lactate was more than 12 mmol/l. Care was withdrawn on day 6 in view of a very poor prognosis.

Cranial ultrasound showed development of increased periventricular echogenicity, more pronounced in the left hemisphere, over the first days. An MRI performed on day 5 showed a mild increase in signal intensity in the basal ganglia and thalami, with a reversed signal intensity of the posterior limb of the internal capsule and a right-sided focal periventricular lesion on the inversion recovery sequence (a). Extensive changes were seen with the DWI, more on the left than the right, involving most of the white matter with relative sparing of the basal ganglia, but involving of the internal capsule, thalami, pulvinar, and hippocampal regions bilaterally (b).

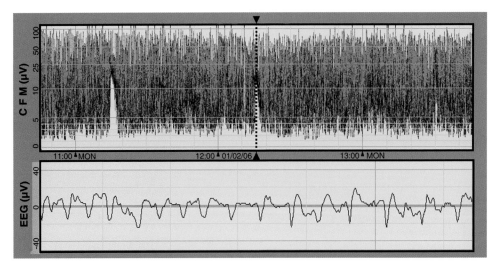

f

Age 67 h.

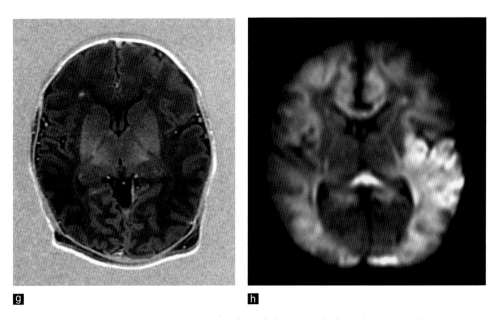

g   **h**

Figure 5.8 *continued*   The aEEG in panel c was started at 6 h, and shows a subclinical status epilepticus ('saw-tooth pattern' in the aEEG) corresponding to irregular sharp and slow wave activity seen on the original EEG. This pattern was interrupted by a loading dose of phenobarbitone (A). The seizures recurred about 1.5 h later and midazolam was started (d) and subsequently lidocaine was added (e). These additional antiepileptic drugs did not have a long-lasting effect and ictal discharges are seen in every panel. The background pattern remained discontinuous over the next couple of days (g and h at 36 and 67 h after birth respectively). A slight recovery from a BS to a discontinuous pattern can be seen in the last panel, recorded 67 h after birth but still showing two ictal discharges. Also note that a mild drift of the baseline (around 5 μV) is seen in panels c–f.

Severe birth asphyxia in the late preterm infant

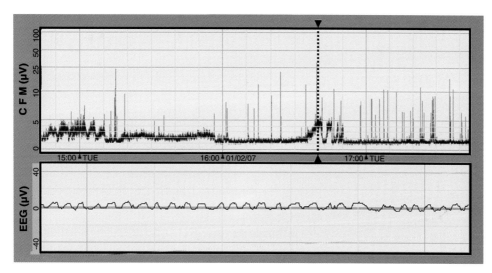

6 h after birth.

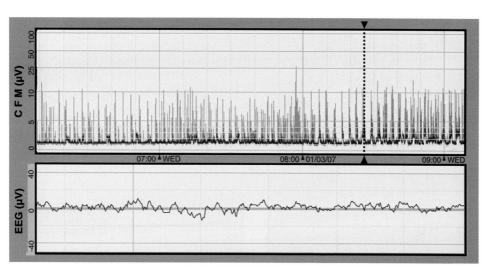

21 h after birth.

Figure 5.9 This female infant was born at 35 weeks' gestation by vaginal breech delivery. She had a poor start and was hand bagged for 20 min until the pediatrician arrived, who intubated and ventilated the infant with rapid recovery of heart rate and spontaneous respiration. The umbilical artery pH was 6.66, with a base excess of –18 mmol/l. The child was referred to the regional NICU where care was withdrawn on day 4 in view of the neuroimaging and neurophysiologic findings.

aEEG was inactive when the registration was started (a). The background pattern remained inactive for the following 6 h, when ictal discharges started to recur (b), and evolved into a prolonged period of status epilepticus which was not initially recognized during the night. Lidocaine was given at about 30 h after birth (B) and was able to stop the status epilepticus (c), and the background pattern became a BS pattern and later again inactive (d).

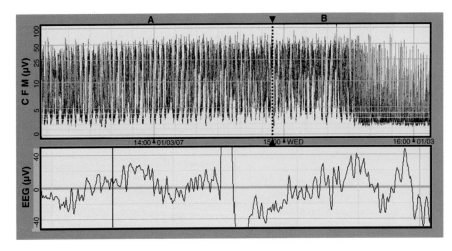

28 h after birth. A, care; B, lidocaine.

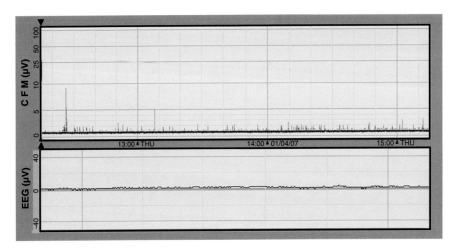

52 h after birth.

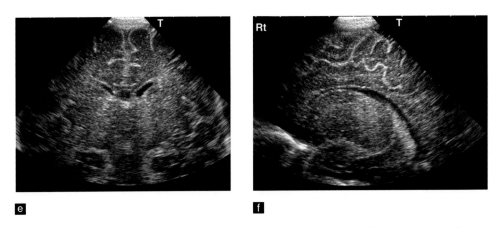

Figure 5.9 *continued* Cranial ultrasound (e) coronal and (f) parasagittal view showed development of severe echogenicity, especially apparent in the basal ganglia, typical of 'acute near total asphyxia'.

This case shows a rather common evolution of the aEEG, starting off with a rather inactive recording, evolving into a BS pattern over the next 12–24 h with ictal discharges, and not uncommonly associated with a status epilepticus. This aEEG also shows that a status epilepticus superimposed on a BS pattern can be missed and interpreted as a BS pattern.

Severe birth asphyxia in a moderately preterm infant

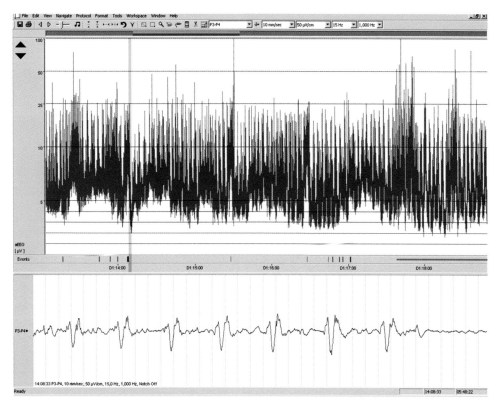

Figure 5.10 This male infant was born after an emergency Cesarean section due to placental abruption at 33 weeks' gestation. His Apgar scores were 0, 2, and 3 at 1, 5, and 10 minutes, respectively. The rescuscitation included administration of epinephrine and sodium bicarbonate, and he was also given surfactant. He developed severe respiratory distress with pulmonary hypertension and was treated with high-frequency ventilation and nitric oxide. He also developed clinical seizures, and received phenobarbitone 10 mg/kg iv. At 9 days of age he was transported to the local hospital in stable condition and early neurodevelopmental outcome at 6 months is good.

MRI was done when he was 4 days old and showed on diffusion-weighted images extensive ischemic lesions, mainly in the parieto-occipital regions and in the basal ganglia.

aEEG was started after arrival at the regional NICU. He had several clinical seizures and the aEEG shows a low-voltage subclinical status epilepticus (note scale for EEG amplitude as compared to other examples) during the 6 h that are shown (a).

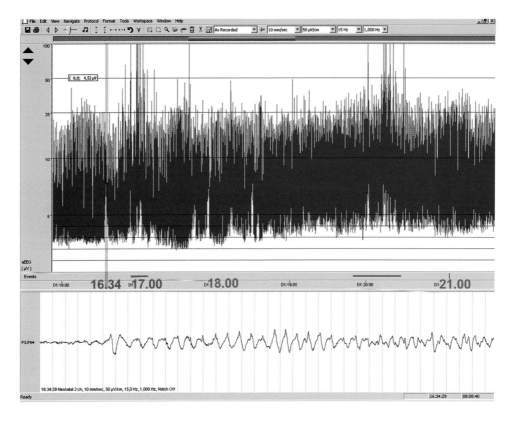

b

Figure 5.10 *continued*   The following day (b) there was a recovery in the aEEG background, but there were still occasional brief seizures at 16:34, before 18:00, and around 18:30. The horizontal green markers below the aEEG around time 17:00 and 21:00 mark care procedures, and there were no seizures during these periods. The small box in the upper left side of the aEEG shows the maximum and minimum aEEG amplitudes at the marker (8.8 and 4.5 μV).

Severe birth asphyxia in a very preterm infant

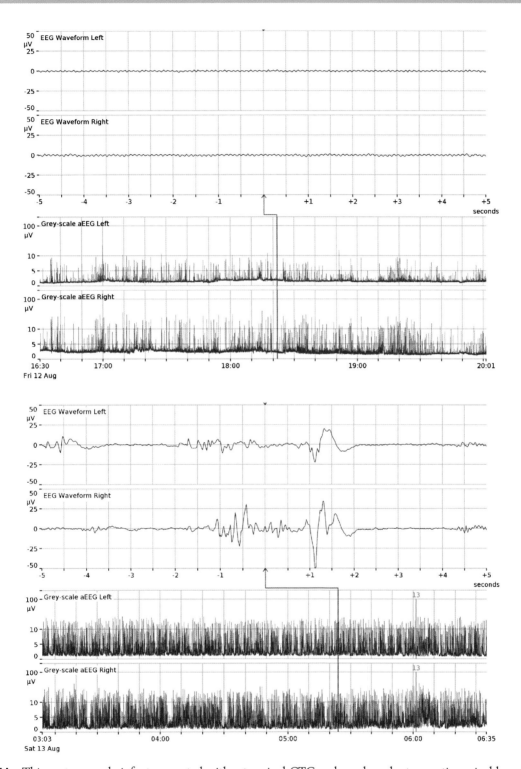

Figure 5.11 This preterm male infant presented with a terminal CTG and was born by traumatic vaginal breech delivery at 30 weeks with a birthweight of 1540 g. His umbilical artery pH was 6.96, with a base excess of –18 mmol/l. He was intubated and ventilated from birth onwards and required inotropic support to maintain adequate blood pressure. Intensive care was withdrawn in view of the poor prognosis.

Cranial ultrasound showed a small intraventricular hemorrhage and periventricular echogenicity, and possibly blood in the posterior fossa. aEEG was started soon after admission and showed an inactive recording (a). Gradual recovery of the background occurred (b).

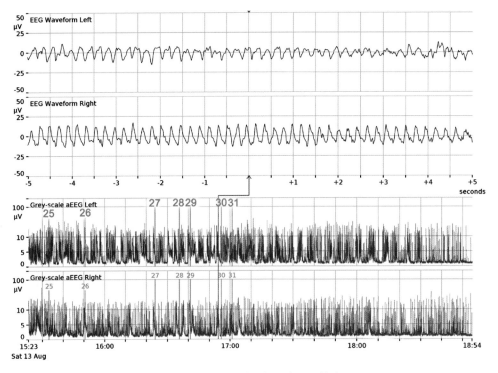

Markers 25: care; 26–29 and 30: high BP; 31: loading dose of lidocaine.

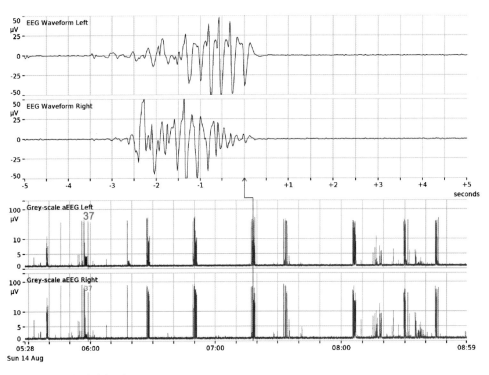

Markers 37: high blood pressure.

Figure 5.11 *continued* Most seizures were subclinical, although many were associated with a rise in blood pressure. Clonazepam was given with little effect (marker 23). Lidocaine was given in (c) (marker 31), when ictal discharges were noted to persist, still more on the left than on the right side. In (d) the recording is mainly inactive, with short bursts of abnormal activity of 2–3 s.

6

Focal hemorrhagic and ischemic lesions in the full-term infant

Newborn infants with seizures but without neonatal encephalopathy are more likely to have focal hemorrhagic or ischemic lesions as an underlying diagnosis.[137] Presentation is usually beyond the first 12 h, in contrast to those with HIE. Hemiconvulsions may initially be the presenting symptom and are further suggestive of a unilateral lesion. In unilateral or asymmetric brain lesions, e.g. middle cerebral artery infarction, unilateral watershed infarction, or a focal parenchymal hemorrhage, concomitant asymmetry of the EEG background activity is common. It has been shown that the EEG background activity over the affected hemisphere is sensitive for prediction of later outcome, a normal background being predictive of normal outcome, while an abnormal background increases the risk that the infant will develop a hemiplegia.[138]

With the introduction of digital aEEG, the use of two channels has become available, enabling the detection of asymmetry in seizure onset and background activity. As cranial ultrasound, performed within the first few days after its onset, will not be able to show increased echogenicity in those with focal infarction, the presence of asymmetry in background activity can suggest a unilateral lesion. In infants where cranial ultrasound does show a unilateral parenchymal hemorrhage, recording with two channels will also be preferable. Even though most unilateral ictal discharges will be detected on the cross-cerebral recording, it is preferable to see in which hemisphere the ictal discharges have their onset. Besides asymmetry in background activity, asymmetry in the presence of sleep–wake cycling can also be seen to occur. During a 10-year period, about 10% of our full-term infants showed a unilateral lesion on neuroimaging.[139]

Background asymmetry due to middle cerebral artery infarction

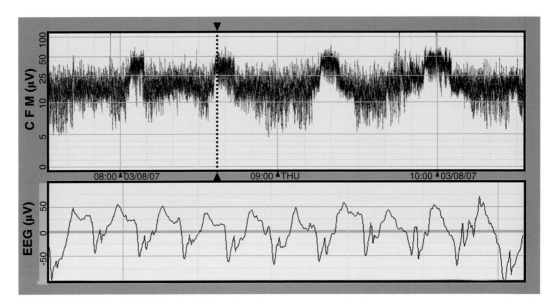

a

16 h after birth.

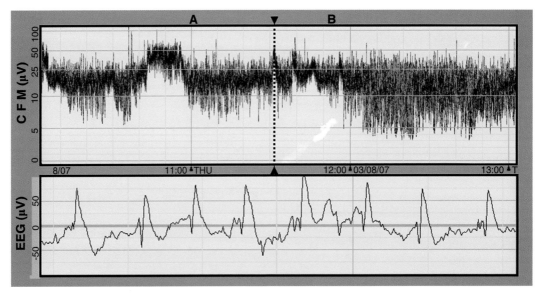

b

EEG done at A–B, three ictal discharges are confirmed arising in the right central region; phenobarbitone loading dose at B.

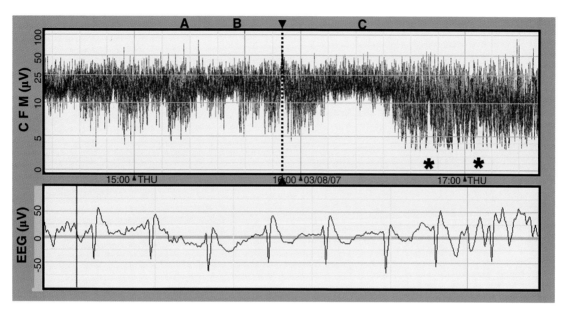

23 h after birth. A, ultrasound; B, care; C, midazolam loading dose.

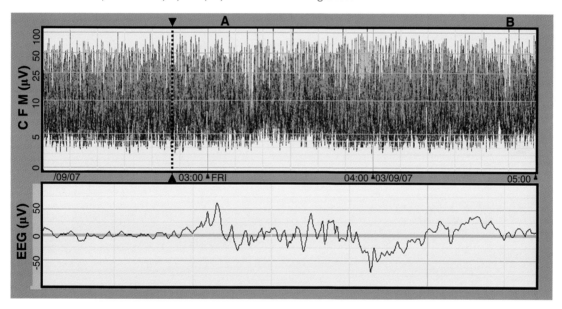

34.5 h after birth. A and B, care.

Figure 6.1 *continued*   This male infant was born at 39 weeks' gestation, birthweight 3500 g, following an unplanned home delivery. After birth he developed grunting and later also apneas, and was intubated and ventilated before transportation to the regional NICU, but required low pressures and minimal oxygen. His initial ultrasound examination on admission was unremarkable, but over the next two days an asymmetry in echogenicity appeared, strongly suggestive of a large right-sided middle cerebral artery infarct. He was never noted to have clinical seizures except for the apneas which occurred a few hours after the delivery. He developed a left-sided hemiplegia.

aEEG monitoring was started with a single-channel monitor, and shows four seizures corresponding to repetitive spike-wave complexes in the EEG below (a). A standard EEG was performed simultaneously with the aEEG (b, beween A and B) and verified the seizure activity seen in the aEEG. The EEG showed that the ictal discharges originated from the right central region. A loading dose of phenobarbitone was given, and resulted in a slightly discontinuous aEEG background and a good initial effect on the seizures (B). Recurrence of ictal discharges was seen a few hours later, and midazolam was added (C), but a few short subclinical seizures are still seen; although not easily recognized in the aEEG they are clearly seen in the EEG (*, c).

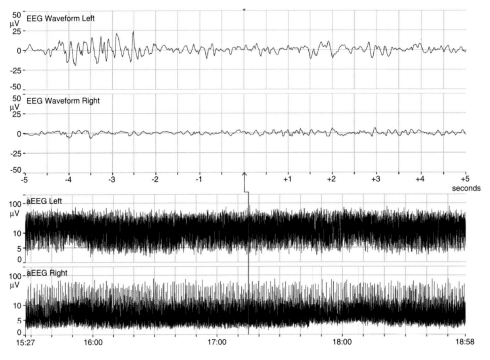

48 h

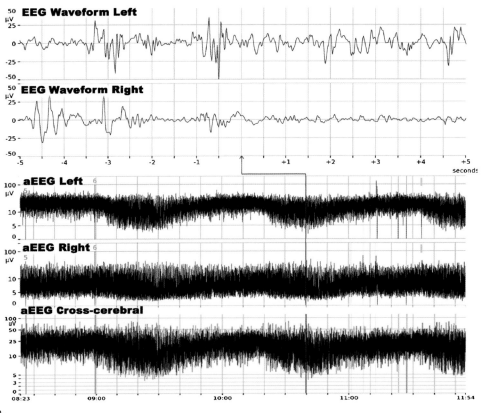

68 h.

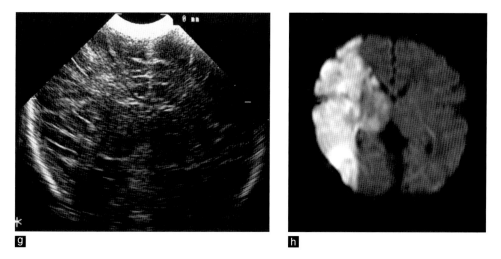

Figure 6.1 *opposite and above*   Following midazolam the aEEG background became discontinuous again, but there are no clear seizures in panel (d), although the original EEG shows a brief (3–4 s) series of sharp waves. After 48 h, bilateral two-channel monitoring was started when a cranial ultrasound showed asymmetric echogenicity, and a second standard EEG also showed an asymmetric background. Panel (e) shows a clear difference between the two hemispheres in background pattern, which is clearly depressed on the right side. The corresponding EEG shows bilateral continuous activity, which is of higher amplitude on the left side. Panel (f), which was recorded when the infant was 68 h, shows development of mature sleep–wake cycling on the left side and a slightly depressed background with some cycling on the right, affected, side. Looking at the simultaneous cross-cerebral (P3–P4) channel, the difference between the two sides is lost and a normal sleep–wake cycling pattern is seen.

Cranial ultrasound on day 3 showed an area of increased echogenicity with a linear demarcation line in the region of the right middle cerebral artery (g). MRI–DWI performed on day 6 confirmed the diagnosis (h).

This case shows that a single-channel EEG displays seizures from a unilateral lesion well. It also shows the added information obtained by bilateral recordings in case there is a unilateral lesion. Even though the ictal discharges will usually also be seen on the single-channel recording, the ictal discharges will be more marked on the affected side and the asymmetry in background pattern may suggest a unilateral lesion.

Middle cerebral artery infarction in a full-term infant

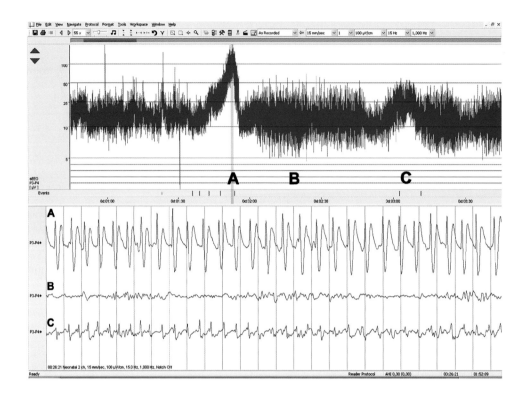

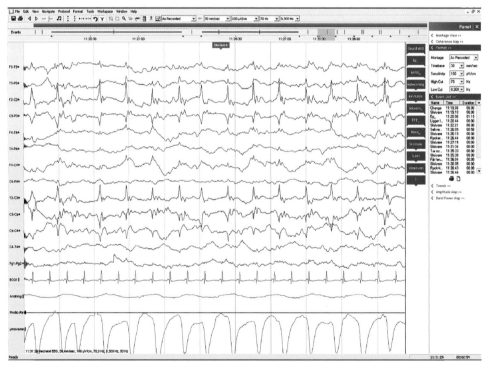

Figure 6.2 This male infant was born at term after a normal pregnancy. During the vaginal delivery the mother developed a fever. He was doing well immediately after birth, and Apgar scores were 9, 10, and 10 at 1, 5, and 10 minutes, respectively. Late in the evening, on the second day after birth, he developed right-sided clonic seizures and was admitted to the NICU. Antiepileptic treatment with phenobarbital, midazolam, and fos-phenytoin was needed to control seizures, but no long-term prophylaxis was given. Outcome at 12 months was normal.

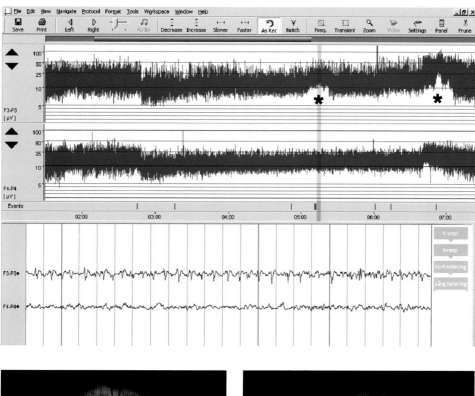

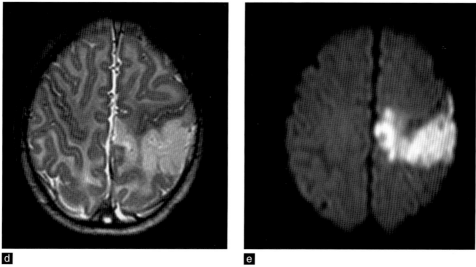

Figure 6.2 *opposite and above* Ultrasound after admission was unremarkable. MRI performed on day 4 showed a cortical branch, middle cerebral artery infarction on the left side, shown with a T_2-weighted spin echo sequence (d) and diffusion-weighted imaging (e).

aEEG was applied as a single-channel recording a quarter before midnight. During the first 2 h there were two electroclinical seizures in the recording (**, a). The EEG shows 25 s of repeated high-voltage sharp-wave activity from the second seizure. The following day a standard EEG was recorded, showing repeated sharp-wave activity over the left hemisphere (b). Due to the asymmetric finding in the EEG, a two-channel aEEG recording was initiated (c). During this 6-h recording two seizures (*) can be identified on the left side (upper aEEG trace). Even though the seizures are clearly identifiable with the two-channel recording, it is quite interesting to note that they are no longer as evident as they were in the single-channel recording. The electrocortical background is still continuous, with some variability but no clear sleep–wake cycling; note the slightly lower aEEG amplitudes (best seen in the lower border of the aEEG traces) over the affected left side.

Intraventricular and intraparenchymal hemorrhage in a full-term infant

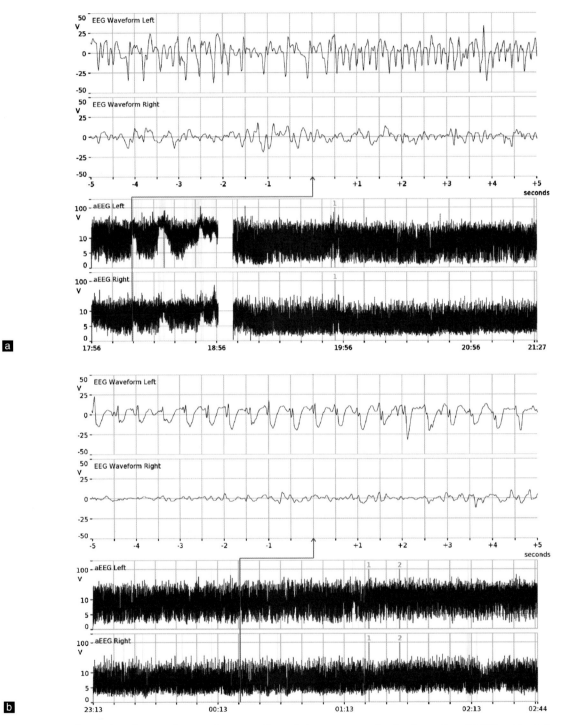

Figure 6.3 This male infant was born at home at 40 weeks' gestation with a birthweight of 3070 g. Fundal expression was used during the last stage of delivery. His Apgar scores were 6, 9, and 10 at 1, 5, and 10 minutes, respectively. He did not feed very well and 24 h after birth two cyanotic episodes were noted. He was taken to hospital, where a large left-sided unilateral intracranial hemorrhage was diagnosed. No underlying etiology was found, and platelet counts were normal. He developed posthemorrhagic ventricular dilatation and eventually required a ventriculo-peritoneal shunt. He was noted to have developed a mild right-sided hemiplegia when last seen at 13 months of age.

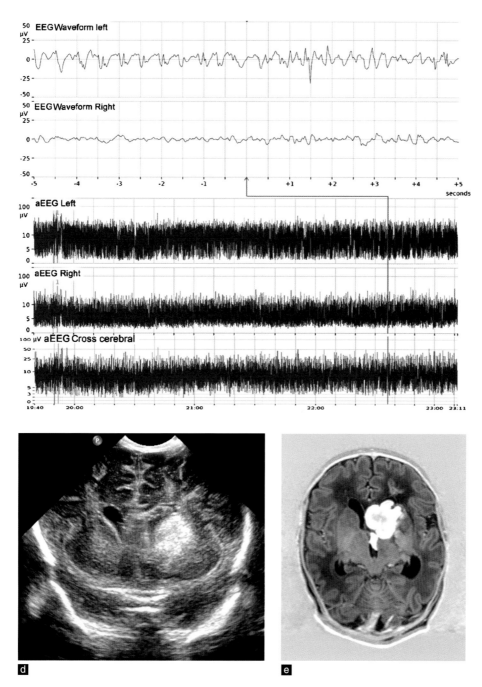

Figure 6.3 *opposite and above*   The aEEG recording was started immediately following admission, using a two-channel recording in view of the ultrasound diagnosis of a unilateral lesion. Several clear ictal discharges are seen at the beginning of the registration, seen most clearly on the left-sided aEEG, confirmed to be irregular spike waves followed by a 7 Hz wave ictal discharge on the original EEG (a). There is no clear difference in the background pattern of the two channels. (b and c) Very short elevations of the trace are seen and these were confirmed to be short 2 Hz spike-wave complexes on the original EEG. It is of interest that these could also be recognized on the cross-over recording. Without simultaneous original EEG, these small interruptions of the background pattern could easily have been overlooked.

A cranial ultrasound scan showed a large IVH with parenchymal involvement on the left (d). An MRI (inversion recovery sequence) confirmed the large left-sided intraventricular hemorrhage as well as the parenchymal involvement (e).

This example shows the additional information obtained with two channels in an infant with a predominantly unilateral lesion. It also shows the value of having a simultaneous original EEG of these two channels, as some of the ictal discharges were short and of rather low voltage and could easily be overlooked when only the aEEG would have been available.

Asymmetric seizures in unilateral watershed infarction

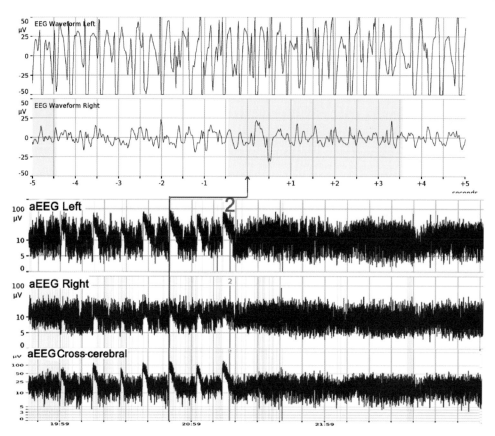

Figure 6.4 This female infant was born at 41 weeks with a birthweight of 3420 g. The delivery was by ventouse extraction and the amniotic fluid was meconium-stained. The Apgar scores were 6 and 8 at 1 and 5 minutes, respectively, and the umbilical artery pH 7.06. She initially went to the postnatal ward and then home a few hours later. Following discharge she developed right-sided hemiconvulsions during the first day after birth. She did not require any ventilatory support while treated with antiepileptic drugs and showed a fast recovery. Her neurodevelopmental outcome was well within the normal range when last seen at 18 months with a DQ of 102 (Griffiths assessment developmental scale).

Her aEEG after admission, using two channels, showed seven ictal discharges, each with a duration of 2 to 5 min ('saw-tooth pattern' during the first 1.5 h of recording). The seizures were clearly identifiable in both channels, but they were more evident on the affected left side. All the initial seizures were also seen on the cross-cerebral recording. Lidocaine was given at marker 2 (a). The overall background pattern was mainly continuous, although on the left side it tended to be slightly discontinuous. There is some variability in the background, although not fully developed sleep–wake cycling. The second panel (gray scale) is taken through a period of suspected left-sided short ictal discharges (b).

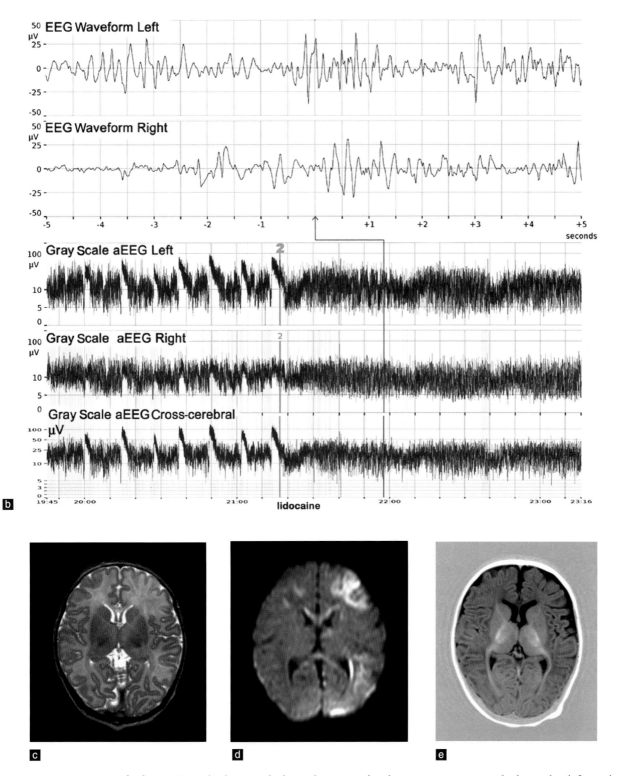

Figure 6.4 *opposite and above* Cranial ultrasound showed increased echogenicity, more marked on the left, and a subsequent MRI, performed on day 6, showed watershed injury, mainly on the left side and more in the anterior watershed region between the anterior and middle cerebral arteries. (c: T_2 spin echo sequence; d: DWI in the neonatal period; e: inversion recovery sequence at 3 months).

Asymmetric ictal discharges in unilateral lobar hemorrhage

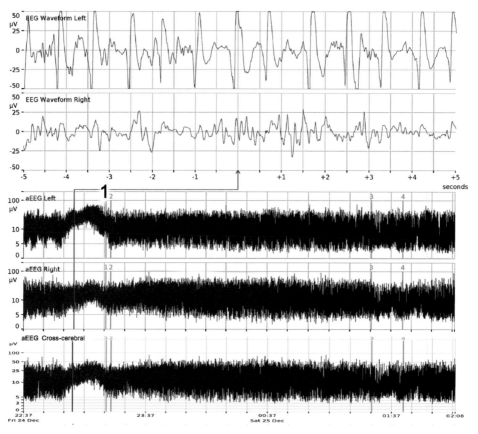

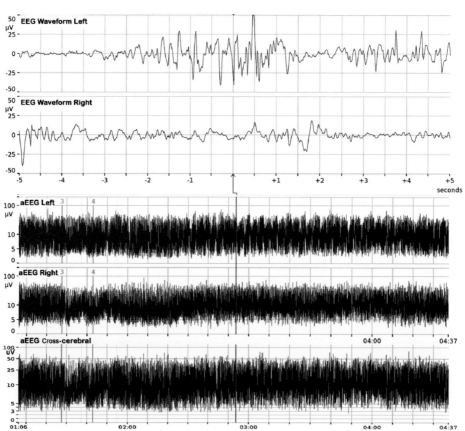

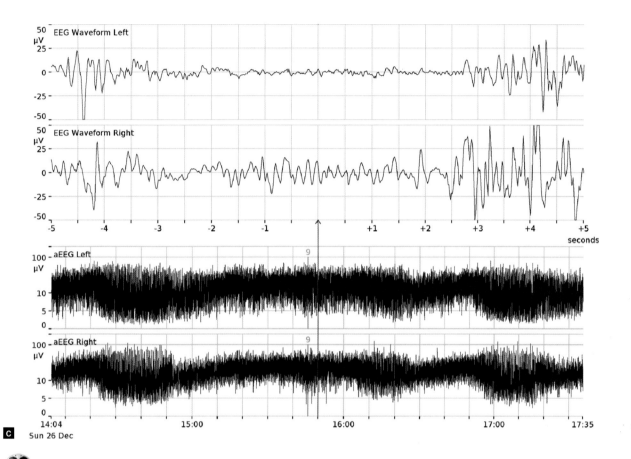

Figure 6.5 *opposite and above*   This female infant was born at 38 weeks' gestation with a birthweight of 2995 g. The delivery was induced because of maternal HELLP syndrome (maternal hemolytic anemia elevated liver enzymes and low platelet count) syndrome, and the child was delivered using ventouse extraction. Her Apgar scores were 8 and 9 at 1 and 5 minutes, respectively. She was pale and hypotonic after birth, and became cyanosed during her first period of breastfeeding, following which she was admitted to the NICU. Neuroimaging showed a subdural hematoma which was surgically removed. Her development was within normal limits at the age of 3 years with a DQ of 95 (Griffiths assessment developmental scale), but with signs of a verbal dyspraxia.

aEEG was recorded following the neurosurgical procedure, the initial aEEG background was continuous (a). After 20 min a prolonged elevation of the aEEG background, most marked on the recording from the left hemisphere as well as on the cross-cerebral recording (P3–P4), occurred. The simultaneous EEG confirmed this to be a prolonged ictal discharge (20 min). A loading dose of midazolam was given at marker 1, followed by a continuous infusion (marker 2); after this a slight depression of the aEEG background is seen, although the EEG is still continuous. (b) An irregular lower margin is seen, suggestive of short ictal discharges; the corresponding EEG showed brief (7–8 s) runs of sharp waves indicative of short seizures on the left side. This is not as clearly seen on the cross-over recording as on the left side, and it is not seen on the right side. There is still a clear difference between the traces from the two hemispheres. The cross-over recording taken during this period shows a discontinuous pattern, although with normal voltage. (c) A good recovery with a continuous voltage pattern and sleep–wake cycling was seen on day 3.

Cranial ultrasound on admission showed a large, left-sided frontal intraparenchymal hematoma and a subdural hematoma associated with a midline shift (d). A CT scan confirmed the midline shift (e), which was the reason to evacuate the subdural collection by an open neurosurgical procedure. An MRI was performed at one week of age, still showing the large parenchymal hematoma as well as an area of high signal intensity surrounding the hematoma on the T_2 spin echo sequence (f) and the diffusion-weighted sequence (g). A repeat scan at 3 months of age shows ex-vacuo enlargement of the left ventricle and an area of cavitation in the left frontal lobe (h).

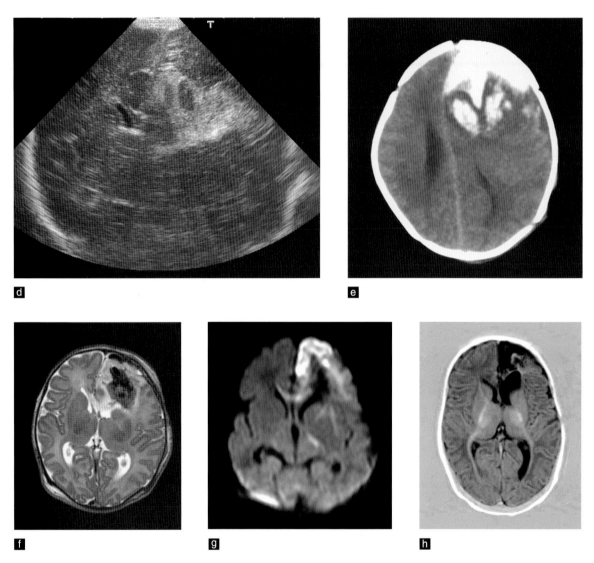

Figure 6.5 *continued*

Asymmetric ictal discharges in unilateral parenchymal hemorrhage

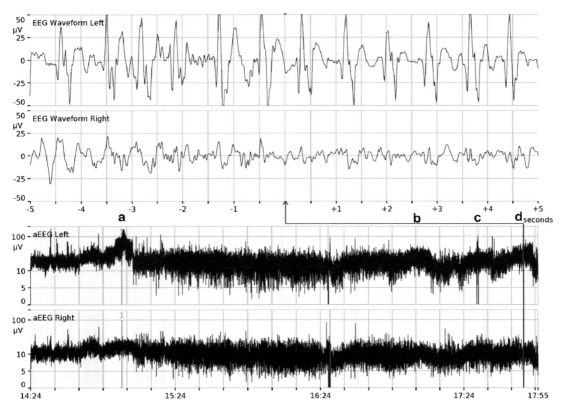

Figure 6.6 This male infant was born at 37 weeks by ventouse extraction and weighed 2540 g. His Apgar scores were 8 and 8 at 1 and 5 minutes, respectively. He was grunting and required oxygen; a chest X-ray showed a left-sided tension pneumothorax and a chest drain was inserted. The following day he was noted to have right-sided jerking movements of his right hand and was referred to the regional NICU for suspected seizures. He was discharged home after one week. He was seen at 24 months; at that time he had developed a very mild right-sided hemiplegia and had a DQ of 98.

(a) The aEEG registration was started when the right-sided clinically suspected seizures had occurred. The initial part of the recording shows a left-sided slow rise of the aEEG trace, which reaches a maximum after 40 min from the start of the recording. This was confirmed by the original EEG to be a left-sided ictal discharge. In the latter part of the trace there are three periods with rather mild elevation of the baseline, each with a duration of 15–20 min with a slow and sustained rise. These changes did not look like an ictal discharge in the aEEG, but were recognized as such on the simultaneous original EEG in the left channel. The overall background was of normal continuous voltage. Another ictal discharge is seen in panel (b), again more marked on the left recording. Two periods of artifact are seen in the second part of this panel.

Cranial ultrasound, coronal view angling backwards (b), showed an area of increased echogenicity in the left hemisphere, which was subsequently confirmed on MRI to be a hemorrhage (left sagittal T2-weighted image, c, and axial inversion recovery centrum semiovale, d), which subsequently evolved into a single cyst on the repeat MRI at 3 months (e).

This example shows the importance of having the original EEG on line, which detected the ictal discharges that were not typical in the aEEG, since they did not present with the more common acute rise of the trace, but instead as slow, sustained, and moderate increases, and the decreases of the aEEG amplitude.

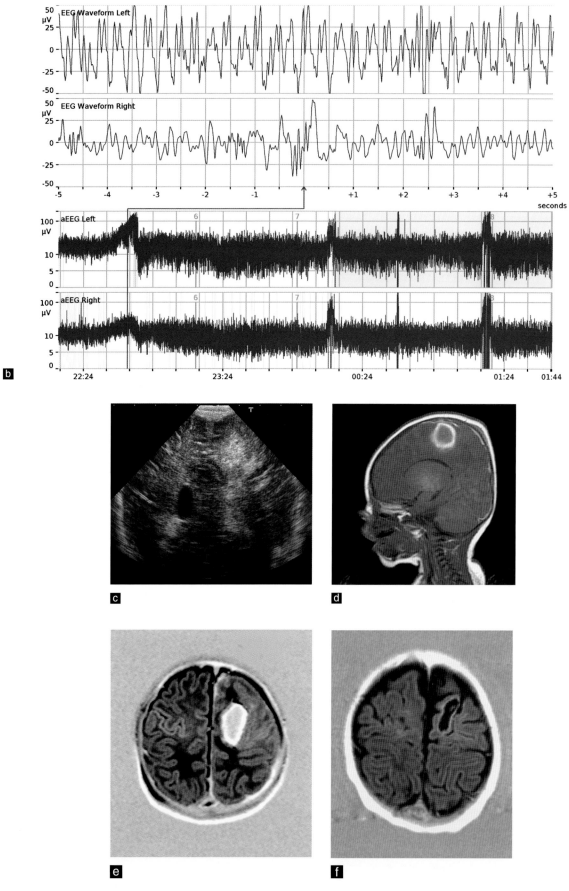

Figure 6.6 *continued*

Asymmetry in background due to subdural hematoma

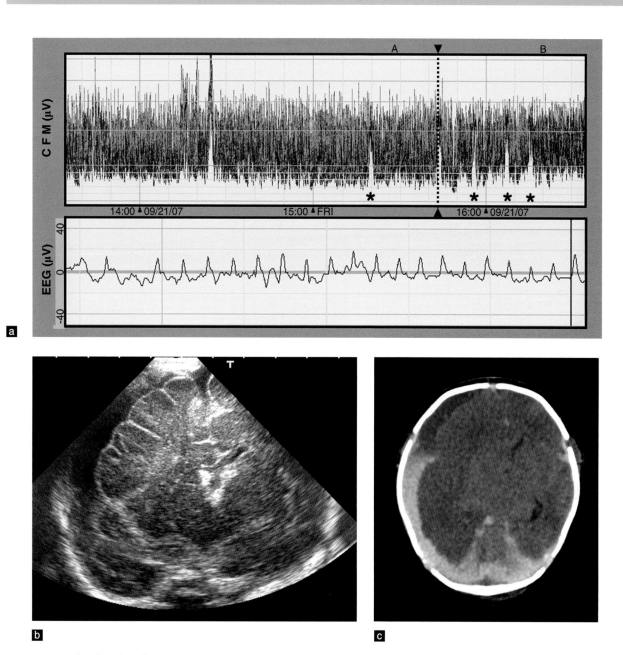

Figure 6.7   This female infant was born at 38 weeks' gestation with a birthweight of 2995 g. An emergency Cesarean section was performed due to placental abruption with fetal bradycardia (50 beats/min) for a period of at least 20 min. Her Apgar scores were 8 and 9 at 1 and 5 minutes, respectively. Neuroimaging was unremarkable on admission but showed a large subdural hematoma at 24 h of age, associated with severely delayed APTT (78 s) and prothrombin time of 36 s. No neurosurgical procedure was done in view of the coagulopathy and her history, and she died shortly afterwards.

aEEG was initially recorded with a single-channel aEEG (a) and showed a discontinuous pattern with seizure activity (*), when the child was almost 24 h old. Phenobarbitone (20 mg/kg iv) was given at B. Following a repeat ultrasound examination, which showed the right-sided subdural hematoma, a two-channel recording was started, showing burst-suppression with a marked asymmetry and (d) suppression of the aEEG background on the right side. (e) Shows continuing asymmetry and further deterioration of the aEEG background on both sides, now with a sparse burst-suppression pattern.

Cranial ultrasound on admission was unremarkable, but the scan at 24 h, showed a large, right-sided subdural hematoma associated with a midline shift and small bilateral intraventricular hemorrhages (b). A CT scan confirmed the midline shift (c).

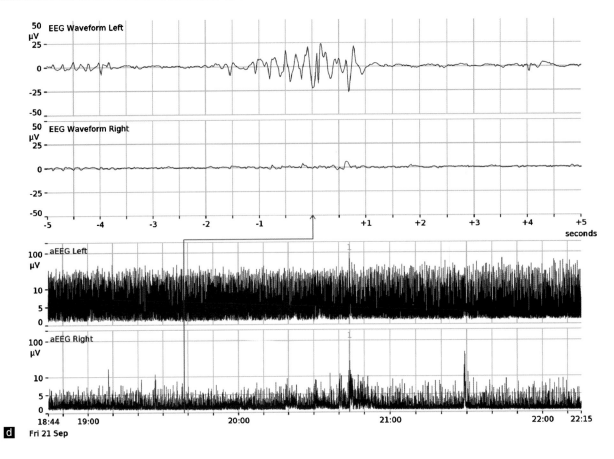

d   Fri 21 Sep

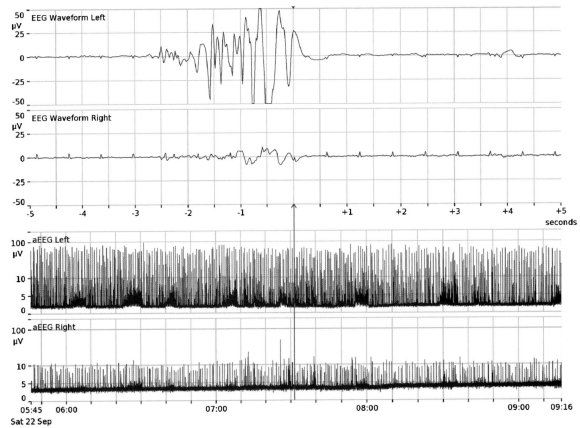

e   Sat 22 Sep

Figure 6.7 *continued*

7

Hemorrhagic and ischemic lesions in the preterm infant

The incidence of germinal matrix/intraventricular hemorrhages (GMH-IVH grades 1–3) and hemorrhagic parenchymal infarction in very preterm infants is decreasing as a result of increased use of antenatal steroids and other improvements in neonatal care. GMH-IVHs are often graded according to the classification by Papile, which will be used in this chapter, although the grade 4 'intraparenchymal hemorrhage' is now usually referred to as periventricular hemorrhagic infarction or venous infarction.[140]

The incidence of focal periventricular ischemic lesions resulting in periventricular cysts, or cystic periventricular leukomalacia (cPVL), is also decreasing. As focal cPVL is uncommon, the term periventricular white matter injury (PWMI) is now more often used.[141] Increased use of MRI techniques and studies performed on preterm infants at term equivalent age have revealed the complex spectrum of white matter damage, which includes punctate white matter lesions (PWMLs) and diffuse excessive high-signal intensity (DEHSI) as well as abnormal structural and functional development.[142] The etiology of white matter damage is multifactorial and important contributors are hypoxic–ischemic injury, excitotoxicity, perinatal infection, and inflammation.

ACUTE STAGE ABNORMALITIES AND BRAIN INJURY IN PRETERM INFANTS

The concept of acute and chronic stage EEG abnormalities is very useful when evaluating EEG in relation to brain injury in both term and preterm infants.[15] Acute stage EEG abnormalities related to hemorrhagic or ischemic lesions in preterm infants are well described and include increased discontinuity, amplitude depression, seizures, and loss of sleep–wake cycling.[15] Early use of EEG can help in identifying acute or established injury.[143] The extent of EEG background abnormalities correlates with the severity of brain damage and with the degree of IVH.[34,50,68,130,144,145] With long-term aEEG monitoring it has also been shown that the duration of EEG background abnormalities is associated with the severity of brain damage and with outcome.[34,37,50] Acute EEG and aEEG changes related to development of cPVL and white matter damage are less well delineated, probably because the time relationship with EEG changes may be difficult to establish, since these lesions are often diagnosed several weeks after the actual insult. However, Connell et al evaluated continuously recorded EEG in relation to parenchymal echodensities on ultrasound (i.e. GMH-IVH and PVL) and observed clear acute stage changes with amplitude depression and seizures.[146] Furthermore, in some studies it was also observed that the EEG background depression sometimes occurred before echodensities appeared on cranial ultrasound.[34,68,146]

CHRONIC STAGE ABNORMALITIES AND BRAIN INJURY IN PRETERM INFANTS

Chronic changes in the EEG related to white matter damage and adverse neurodevelopmental outcome include presence of PRSWs, delayed maturation, and disorganized electrocortical background appearing within weeks after the injury.[147–150] Sleep–wake cycling may also be affected, as shown by EEG power spectral analysis. At term equivalent age there were clear differences between prematurely born infants and full-term infants; the changes were associated with suboptimal cognitive performance.[151] Evaluation of chronic stage abnormalities requires a full standard EEG. Another trend measure of the EEG, the 90% SEF, the EEG frequency below which 90% (or another predefined measure, usually 80 or 90%) of the power in the EEG is distributed, was shown in one study to correlate well with development of white matter damage in preterm infants with a median gestational age of 27 weeks (range 23–31 weeks).[17] Although not formally evaluated as a trend for long-term EEG - monitoring, SEF seems to be a measure that is too sensitive to interference in the NICU to be used for daily clinical monitoring.

PRETERM BRAIN INJURY AND aEEG/EEG CONTINUITY

When early EEG monitoring is applied in very preterm infants, there seems to be an increase in electrocortical activity during the first days of life.[34–36] Whether this is due to transient depression of activity related to birth or an increase triggered by birth itself is not known. However, in infants developing brain damage, the depression is often prolonged.[34] Furthermore, the discontinuous EEG background (tracé discontinu), which is normally seen in the aEEG of very preterm infants as an aEEG pattern with some amplitude variability in the lower border, is often replaced by a BS pattern. The BS is characterized by an unresponsive pattern with a mainly flat (no activity or very low voltage) IBI activity and no cyclicity.

When evaluating the degree of acute brain damage in preterm infants, the background patterns and amplitudes in the aEEG that have been shown to correlate with brain damage in full-term asphyxiated infants cannot be used, due to the discontinuous EEG in normal, very preterm infants. Instead, the IBI, which is a direct measure of continuity in the very preterm EEG and also in the suppressed full-term EEG, can be used. As shown in Chapter 2, the IBI decreases with increasing maturation, but as a 'rule of thumb' the IBI should not be longer than 30–40 s, corresponding to approximately at least 100 bursts/h (the burst count is of course also dependent on the duration of the bursts). An IBI duration of more than 30 s was also shown in term infants with discontinuous EEG to be the EEG feature most closely associated with adverse later outcome.[126]

Studies in pediatric populations indicate that hydrocephalus is associated with an increased amount of slow activity, discontinuity, and asynchrony in the EEG, as well as epileptiform activity.[152,153] The effect of posthemorrhagic ventricular dilatation on EEG has not been systematically investigated in preterm infants, although aEEG data from two preterm infants with progressive hydrocephalus have been published.[154] Increasing hydrocephalus was associated with increased discontinuity and lack of sleep–wake cycling. The aEEG abnormalities were reversible in one of the infants when intracranial pressure was reduced after insertion of a shunt.

PRETERM BRAIN INJURY AND SEIZURES

Earlier studies using conventional EEG, EEG monitoring, or aEEG showed that seizures, often entirely subclinical or with only subtle clinical manifestations, were common during the first days of life in infants developing IVH or PVL.[34,37,50,68,143] In two prospectively evaluated cohorts of preterm infants (mean gestational ages 28 and 26 weeks, respectively) who had early aEEG recorded during the late 1980s, suspected seizures were present during the first days of life in around 65 to 75% of infants developing IVH.[34,37] The expression of seizures in preterm infants developing IVH was quite variable: in some infants only a few single seizures were noted while others developed status epilepticus. The effect of 'seizure burden' on neurologic outcome was not evaluated in these studies. However, in a later study the amount of seizures did not affect outcome in very preterm infants who survived with IVH 3–4.[50] Although not specifically evaluated in modern cohorts of preterm infants, it is our impression that epileptic seizures are less common in preterm infants developing IVH. This impression could, of course, also be due to the lower incidence of IVH in these infants.

PREDICTION OF OUTCOME

Early prediction of outcome from aEEG/EEG is more uncertain in preterm infants than in full-term asphyxiated infants since the degree of prematurity and other related, but primarily non-neurologic, problems may influence neurodevelopmental outcome.[23] However, the early electrocortical background does also contain predictive information in very preterm infants. In preterm infants with GMH-IVH 3–4 it was shown that the maximum number of bursts per hour in the aEEG during the first 48 h of life correlated with outcome.[50] Infants who could produce at least one hour with more than 130 bursts had a 70–80% chance of surviving with no or moderate handicap, as compared to infants with lower burst density, who were more likely to die or survive with severe handicap. The hour including the lowest burst count, i.e. 'minimum bursts/h' was also evaluated but did not have the same sensitivity as the maximum bursts/h, probably because administration of several medications, e.g. morphine and sufentanil, is associated with transient background depression and consequently this measure does not only reflect brain damage. The cut-off at 130 bursts/h cannot be directly used, since the study was retrospective and most infants received phenobarbitone. The reason why bursts were counted in this study, instead of estimating IBI, was that bursts are more easily defined in the old aEEG/CFM without an original EEG display.

Until recently, estimations of IBI had to be performed manually – a cumbersome and time-consuming process. Automated calculation of IBI is currently developed in some of the EEG monitors (see Figure 1.10a). There are several issues that have to be considered when estimating IBI in EEG; the most important are the cut-off levels when activity should be classified as IBI or as 'burst', especially in the preterm EEG where the IBI is not flat but contains low-amplitude activity.[155] Normative data of IBI, from manual evaluation of EEG traces, have also used slightly different definitions of IBI.[26–30] However, preliminary data from a cohort of extremely preterm infants, evaluating automated averaged IBI from the first days of life, show that this measure correlates with brain damage and outcome at 2 years.[32]

The predictive value of seizures in the aEEG/EEG in relation to outcome was only investigated in infants with large GMH-IVHs, and in these infants it was not associated with outcome.[50]

Sleep–wake cycling which was present during the first week of life was associated with better outcome in preterm infants with large IVHs.[37,50] The presence of sleep–wake cycling in the aEEG is also associated with good outcome in extremely preterm infants with smaller or no intraventricular hemorrhages.[37,38]

SUMMARY

- The aEEG/EEG at all gestational ages should normally contain at least 100 bursts/h.

- aEEG/EEG changes associated with hemorrhagic or ischemic brain damage in preterm infants include:

   o Increased discontinuity, i.e. increased IBI and/or decreased amplitude (voltage) during the IBI (i.e. BS pattern instead of *tracé discontinu*);

   o Presence of epileptic seizure activity, often subclinical;

   o Loss of sleep–wake cycling;

   o Recovery within 1–2 weeks, chronic stage changes may persist and are best evaluated with standard EEG.

Mild white matter injury in preterm infant with esophageal atresia and pneumothorax

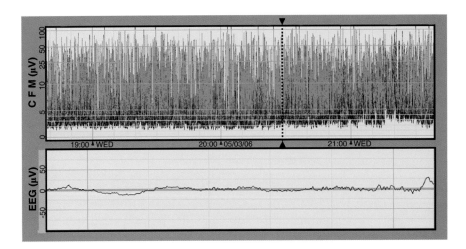

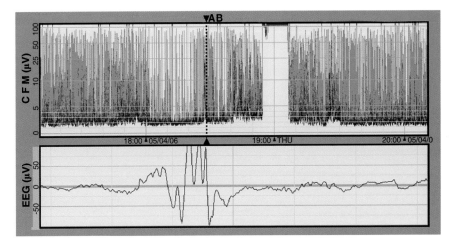

A, surfactant; puncture pneumothorax; B, drain insertion pneumothorax.

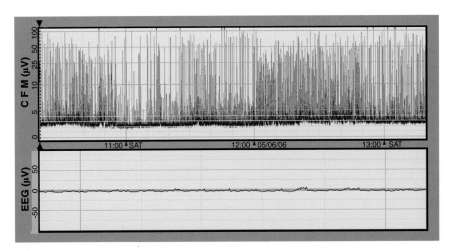

Day 4.

Figure 7.1 This male infant was born at 32 weeks' gestation by emergency Cesarean section due to placental abruption. His birthweight was 1700 g. Antenatal ultrasound suggested esophageal atresia, which was confirmed following delivery. He had surgery on day 2, and had a complicated postoperative course including a pneumothorax with very high arterial (100 mmHg) pCO_2 values. There was a global delay when he was seen at 18 months of age.

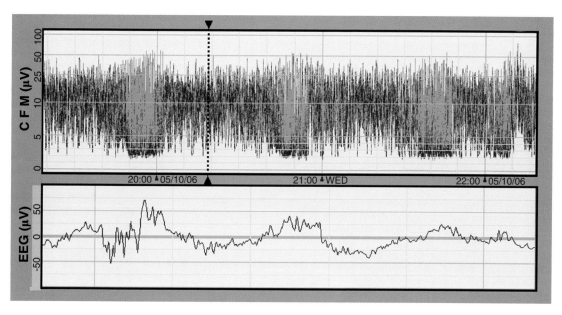

d

Day 8.

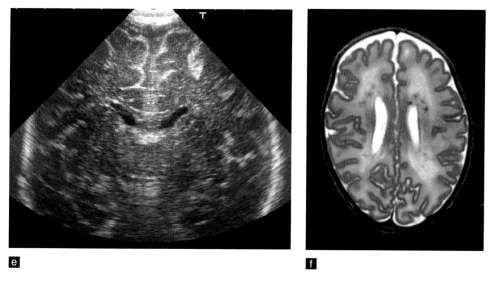

e   f

Figure 7.1 *opposite and above* aEEG showed a discontinuous pattern with little variation, which is acceptable in this preterm infant who is ventilated and receiving morphine as sedation (a). In (b), at 18:00h, a rather abrupt decrease in burst density is seen, when the infant develops a tension pneumothorax with high pCO_2 levels, but without associated hypotension or hypoxemia. The burst density increases following insertion of a pleural drainage. Panel (c) initially shows a BS pattern with very sparse burst density, including IBIs of several minutes' duration; the burst density increases at the end of the trace but is still clearly abnormal. The corresponding EEG from 11.00 during an IBI is flat but contains ECG artifacts. When he is a week old, normal sleep–wake cycling for a moderately preterm infant is seen (d).

Cranial ultrasound showed persistent periventricular echogenicity but no subsequent cystic evolution (PVL grade 1). The widening of the interhemispheric fissure is well seen on the US at term equivalent age (e) and the term equivalent MRI (f) showed diffuse excessive high signal intensity of the white matter on a T2SE sequence as well as punctate white matter lesions and widening of the extracerebral space.

Preterm infant with a small GMH-IVH with seizures and suspect outcome

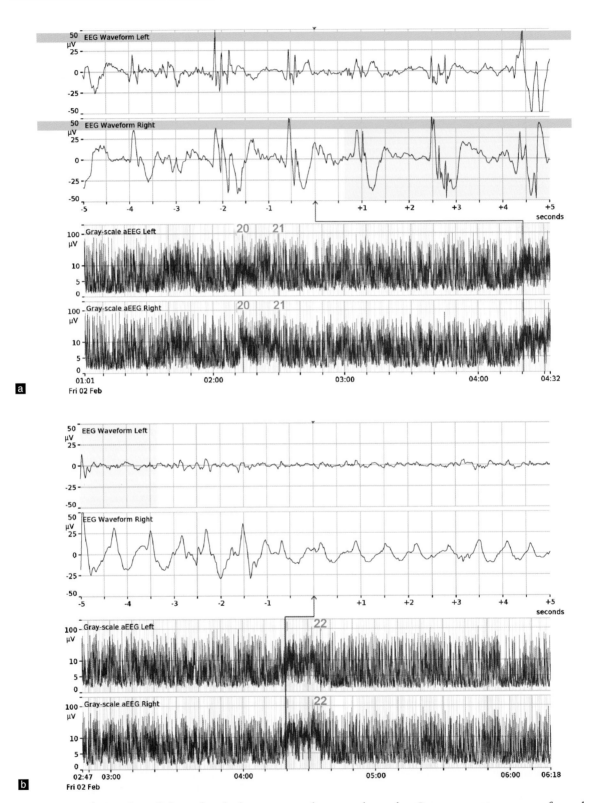

Figure 7.2 The mother of this infant had a severe cardiomyopathy and a Cesarean section was performed when the mother's condition deteriorated. This male infant was born at 27 weeks' gestation, with a birth weight of 1130 g. His Apgar scores were 3, 6, and 6 at 1, 5, and 10 minutes, even though he was immediately intubated and ventilated. He developed RDS and required high-frequency ventilation and surfactant. His early development at 6 months was mildly abnormal.

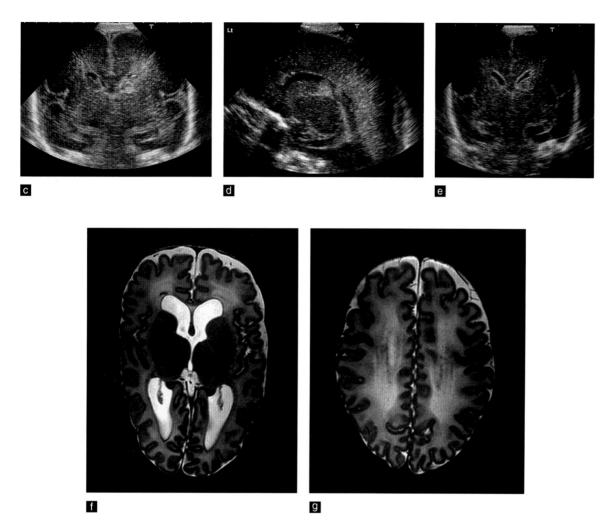

Figure 7.2 *opposite and above*   aEEG recording was started when he was a week old and developed unexplained bradycardias, while he was still on the ventilator. He developed electroclinical as well as electrographic seizures. Panel (a) shows a rather disorganized and discontinuous-looking aEEG pattern with an ictal discharge recognized with the seizure detection ('EEG waveform') showing sharp and slow wave complexes of 1–1.5 seconds' duration in the original EEG. Another ictal discharge was recognized by the automatic seizure detection in (b), showing sharp and slow wave complexes of 0.7 Hz. Care was given at marker 21 and lidocaine at marker 22.

Cranial ultrasound on admission showed a small left-sided IVH associated with periventricular echogenicity (c, d). Mild ventriculomegaly developed later on ultrasound (e), and is also seen on the term age equivalent MRI-T2 weighted spinecho sequence (f), associated with diffuse high signal intensity, best seen at the level of the centrum semiovale (g).

This case shows the additional value of the aEEG for diagnosing seizures in a preterm infant with subtle clinical symptoms, mainly apneas which occurred rather suddenly and unexpectedly after one week and could not be explained by late onset infection. There was an unexplained discrepancy between the severity of the seizures documented on the aEEG and the small hemorrhage with mild periventricular echogenicity seen on cranial US.

Preterm infant with bilateral GMH-IVH

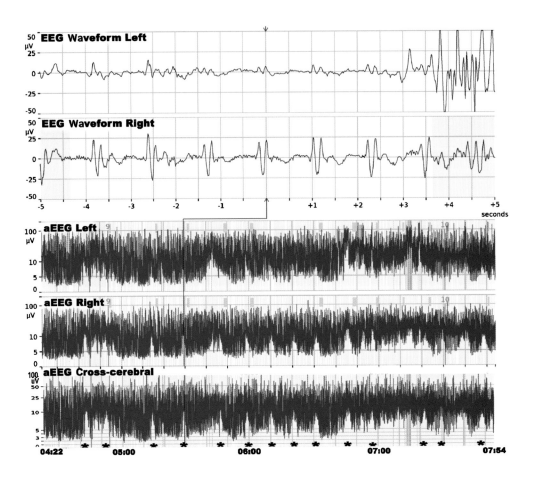

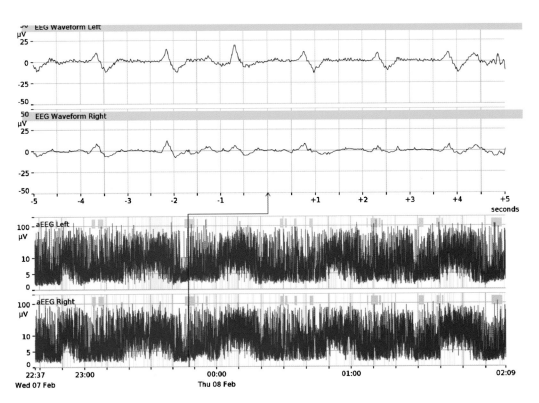

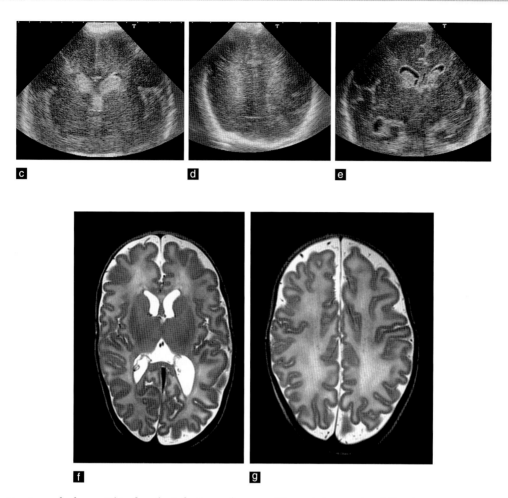

Figure 7.3 *opposite and above* This female infant was born at 29 weeks' gestation following premature rupture of the membranes, and her mother developed fever before the vaginal delivery. Her birthweight was 1200 g. Apgar scores were 8 and 9 at 1 and 5 minutes, respectively. The initial arterial lactate was 7.8 mmol/l. C-reactive protein (CRP) was 57 mg/l, but all cultures remained negative. She developed grunting after birth and required continuous positive airway pressure (CPAP). She survived but long-term outcome is not yet known; however, she was doing very well at 12 months corrected age.

In view of the early diagnosis of the IVH, the aEEG was started immediately. While the quality of the initial background pattern is difficult to evaluate due to repetitive subclinical seizures, it looks slightly depressed and 'unorganized' for the GA, although it has some variability and a rather dense burst pattern (a). The seizures are more marked over the right hemisphere, in spite of similar amounts of blood in both lateral ventricles. However, the right-sided dominance of seizures fits well with the cranial ultrasound scan, which showed more periventricular echogenicity on the right side. A cross-over recording also clearly shows the ictal discharges and a considerable number were recognized with the seizure detection (orange blocks). Most of the ictal discharges are marked (*). They were confirmed with the original EEG as sharp and slow wave complexes of 1.5 seconds' duration. Seizures persisted for more than one day in spite of phenobarbitone therapy. In (b) the ictal discharges are seen during more discontinuous periods and are not always associated with a clear rise of the lower and upper margin of the background pattern.

Cranial ultrasound performed within 1 h after birth showed a moderate bilateral IVH, both in the mid-coronal view and in the coronal view, angling backwards, and increased echogenicity in the periventricular white matter, more marked on the right side (c) and bilaterally in the coronal view angling backwards (d). The ultrasound taken after 2 weeks shows resolution of the hemorrhage with mild ventricular dilatation (e). The MRI at term equivalent age shows mild changes in the white matter, mild ventriculomegaly, and normal myelination of the posterior limb of internal capsule (PLIC) (f and g).

This case illustrates the fact that seizures, often subclinical, are not uncommon in preterm infants with IVH and white matter injury. Without continuous EEG monitoring they could probably remain unrecognized. The preserved electrocortical background in this infant, with early sleep–wake cycling, is indicative of a relatively good outcome. This case also shows that the simultaneous EEG must be evaluated for brief ictal discharges in preterm infants with a mainly discontinuous EEG background, and that the seizure-detection alert can be helpful to recognize ictal discharges.

Preterm infant with parenchymal hemorrhage and poor outcome

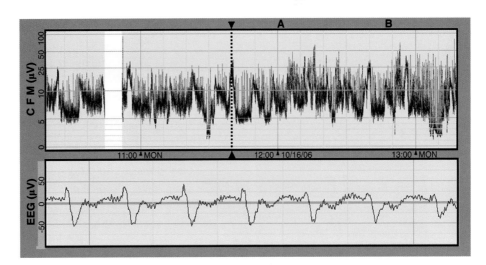

A, EEG; B, lidocaine.

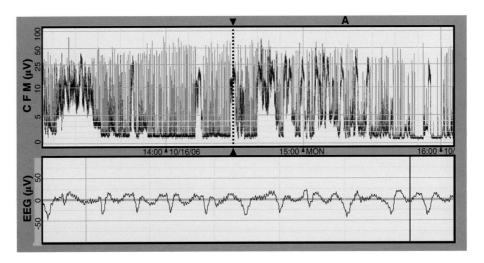

A, clonazepam.

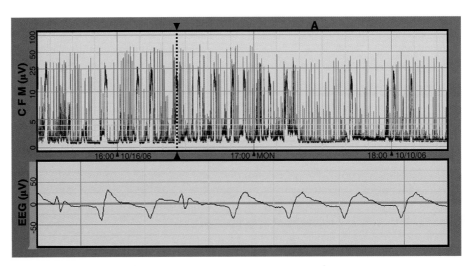

A, clonazepam increased.

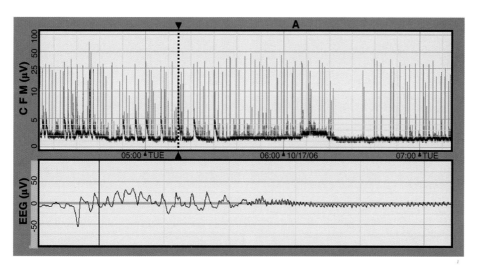

A, phenobarbitone.

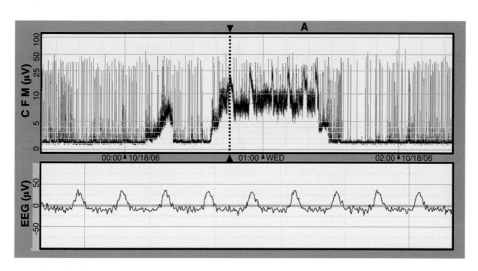

A, phenobarbitone.

Figure 7.4 *opposite and above*   This male infant was the survivor of twin-to-twin transfusion syndrome, treated with laser coagulation at 20 weeks' gestation. He was born at 29 weeks' gestation by vaginal breech delivery following prolonged premature rupture of the membranes. Birth weight was 1440 g, and Apgar scores were 1 and 8, at 1 and 5 minutes, respectively. He needed brief bag and mask ventilation after the delivery, but was coping well with nasal CPAP until 12 h of age, when he developed frequent apneas and required intubation and mechanical ventilation. Cultures from the ear, throat, and umbilical region were all positive for group B streptococci, although the blood culture was negative. The C-reactive protein (CRP) later rose to 88 mg/l. In view of the severe neurologic problems, intensive care therapy was eventually withdrawn.

aEEG was started when the IVH was diagnosed. Subclinical ictal discharges developed within the first 12 h after birth. The seizures were impossible to control, in spite of administration of phenobarbitone, lidocaine, and clonazepam. In (a), recorded 24 h after birth, repetitive ictal discharges are seen on a low-voltage BS pattern on an elevated baseline. The suspected seizures in the aEEG were confirmed with the single-channel EEG below, and with a standard EEG, as sharp and slow-wave complexes of 1.2 s duration. Panels (b) to (e) show persistent subclinical seizures and an increasingly depressed background. The dramatic increase in the IVH occurred between panels (b) and (c). In panel (e), the ictal discharges are again seen during a period of baseline elevation, which is probably caused by external non-cerebral interferences. Fast activity of low amplitude is seen in several panels, but is especially marked in the second part of panel (b). It is not clear what this is due to; similar activity can be caused by high-frequency ventilation and maybe also by the incubator, and should not be confused with seizures.

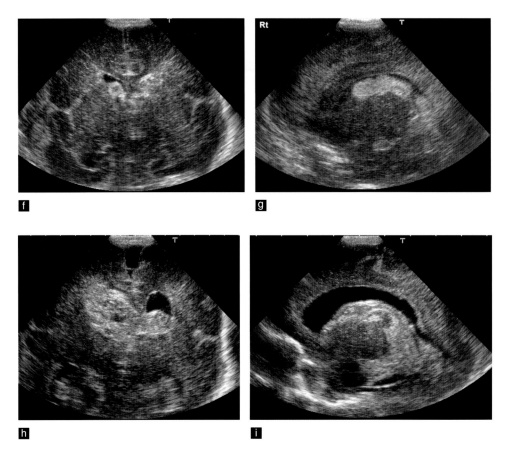

Figure 7.4 *continued*   Cranial ultrasound on admission showed small bilateral intraventricular hemorrhages (f) and (g). The haemorrhages were still small 48 hours later, when prolonged seizures had been going on for more than 24 h. The hemorrhages then increased in size overnight, with acute ventricular dilatation and associated parenchymal involvement of the right periventricular white matter (h) and (i).

This infant illustrates that cranial ultrasound is not always sufficient to evaluate the severity of brain injury in high-risk infants, and shows the utility of continuous EEG monitoring in such infants. While this infant initially appeared well, and aEEG was only started because of a small IVH, repetitive seizures appeared on a severely abnormal background and were initially associated with apneas. The continuously ongoing seizures preceded the parenchymal hemorrhagic involvement by more than 24 h.

Preterm infant with large GMH-IVH, cerebellar hemorrhage, and poor outcome

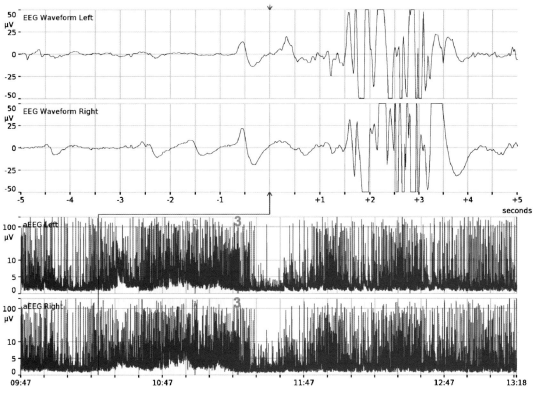

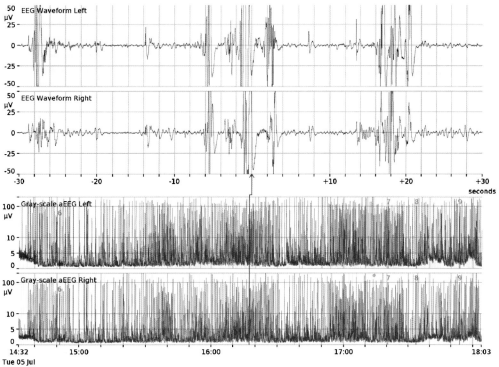

Figure 7.5 This male infant was born at 27 weeks' gestation, with a birthweight of 950 g. An emergency Cesarean section was performed due to placental abruption, Apgar scores were 3 and 9 at 1 and 5 minutes, respectively. He developed severe RDS and needed repeated doses of surfactant. He also required dopamine and dobutamine for arterial hypotension. Intensive care was withdrawn on day 4 in view of the poor prognosis.

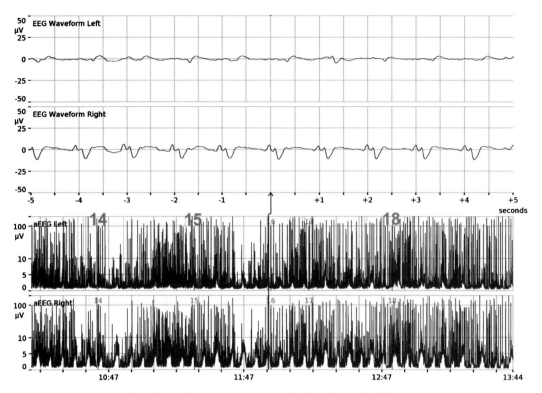

48 h. Markers: 14, loading dose of iv clonazepam; 15, loading dose of iv lidocaine.

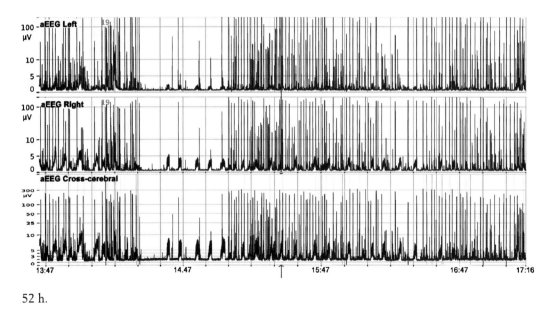

52 h.

Figure 7.5 *continued*   aEEG was started shortly after admission and showed a discontinuous pattern with long IBIs. The lack of variability in the lower aEEG border in (e) indicates that this is a depressed BS pattern and not a *tracé discontinue* background. The abnormal background is also appreciated from the clearly visible bursts, which indicate rather sparse burst activity. This is further emphasized following administration of phenobarbitone (at marker 3) for suspected seizure activity. A few sharp and slow waves precede the bursts in the right EEG recording. The discontinuous pattern as well as the long IBIs, of 14–20 s, are better appreciated in (b), taken with the gray scale, with the original EEG showing 1 min per screen instead of 10 s. In (c), recorded when he was 48 h old, repetitive discharges (sharp and slow-wave complexes of 1/s) can be seen more clearly on the right than on the left tracing, in agreement with the side of the IVH. The original EEG shows that the ictal discharges are of low voltage. Seizures were confirmed on the standard EEG that was recorded between markers 14 and 18.

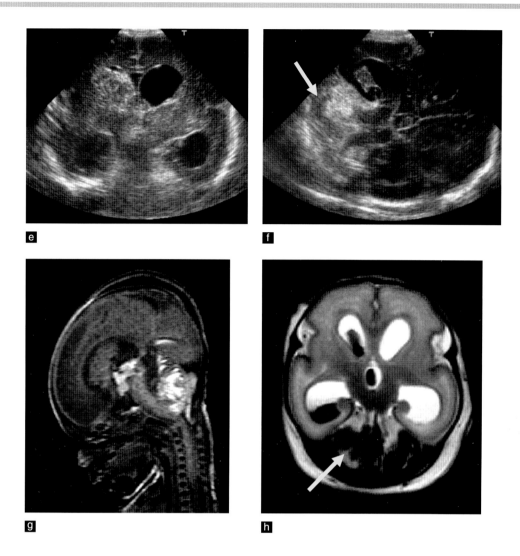

Figure 7.5 *opposite and above*   The seizures were resistant to clonazepam and lidocaine and the background pattern became more depressed. Panel (d) also shows a cross-cerebral (P3–P4) recording which further improved detection of the ictal discharges, which were suspected but were not clear on either the left-side or on the right-side recording (see videoclip).

(e and f) The first cranial ultrasound examination showed only mild periventricular echogenicity. However, on day 2 he had a full fontanelle and a repeat scan showed a large, right-sided IVH as well as a suspected cerebellar hemorrhage, best seen on an axial view through the temporal bone (f, arrow). These findings were subsequently confirmed on day 3 by an MRI (g and h).

A thalamic and intraventricular hemorrhage in a preterm infant with agenesis of the corpus callosum

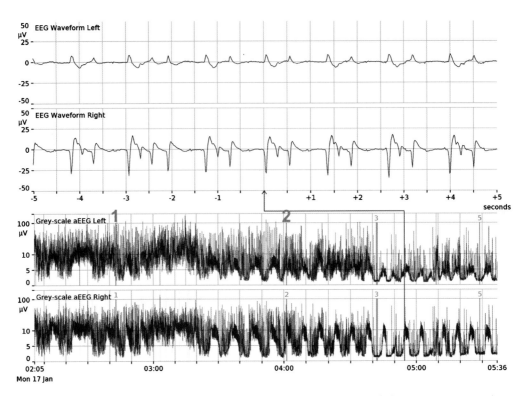

Markers: 1, loading dose of iv phenobarbitone; 2, continuous infusion of clonazepam is started.

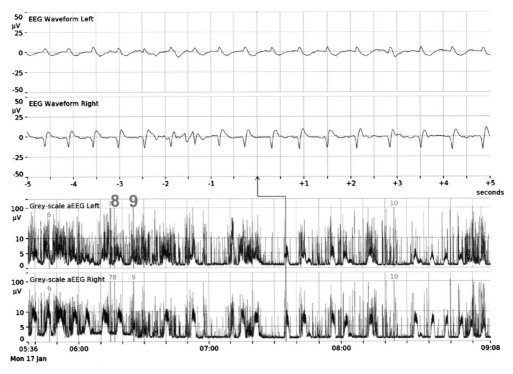

Markers: 8, loading dose of iv lidocaine; 9, second dose of phenobarbitone.

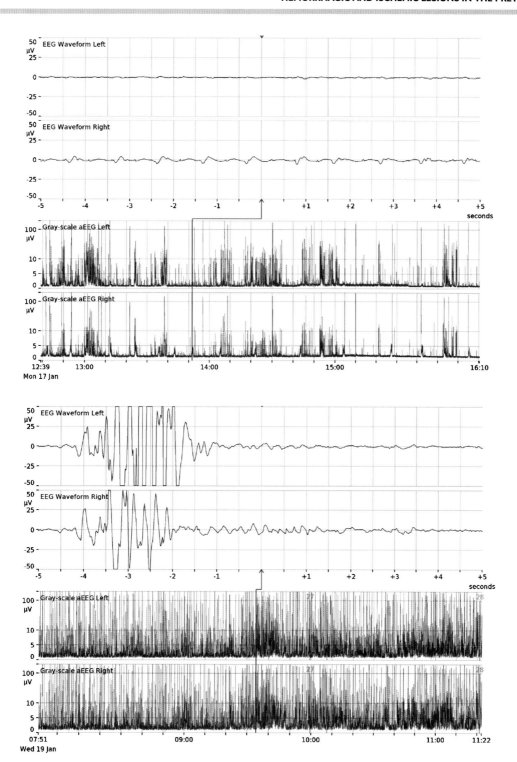

Figure 7.6 *opposite and above*   This male infant was born at 31 weeks' gestation with a birth weight of 1600 g. His Apgar scores were 4, 6, and 7 at 1, 5, and 10 minutes, respectively. The umbilical artery pH was 7.0, with a base excess of −18 mmol/l, and the first arterial lactate was 7 mmol/l. An antenatal MRI had already shown ventricular dilatation and agenesis of the corpus callosum.

He was initially on nasal CPAP, but developed apneas during the first 12 hours after birth and required ventilation until intensive care was withdrawn in anticipation of a poor neurologic outcome.

The aEEG recording was started when the apneas presented, and revealed repetitive seizures. A loading dose of phenobarbitone (20 mg/kg iv) was given with no major effect on the seizures, and was followed by administration of clonazepam 1 h and 20 min later, as shown in (a). The aEEG background became more depressed after clonazepam, but the ictal discharges persisted and were especially prominent on the right side, which was also the side of the large hemorrhage.

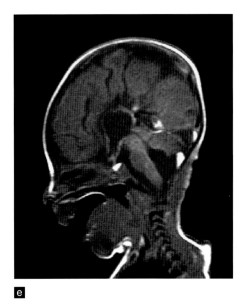

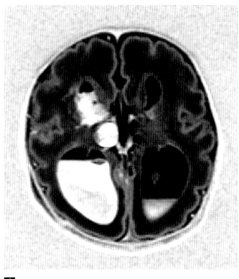

Figure 7.6 *continued*   Panel (b) shows further depression of electrocortical activity, probably as a result of added antiepileptic medications, since a loading dose of lidocaine was given followed by another dose of phenobarbitone. Seizures were eventually controlled, but the electrocortical background was almost flat (inactive). Some very low-voltage discharges can still be recognized with the aEEG and confirmed with the original EEG (c). The last panel (d), recorded on day 4, shows a slight increase in bursts, but the BS background is still very depressed (see videoclip).

Cranial ultrasound and later MRI confirmed the antenatal diagnosis of the agenesis of the corpus callosum, as well as a rotated and small cerebellar vermis. In addition, a large hemorrhage was seen in the right thalamus and in the right lateral ventricle. Some blood was also seen in the left lateral ventricle (e: midsagittal T1-weighted image, f: axial inversion recovery sequence).

This case shows the additional information obtained by the aEEG in an infant who develops repetitive apneas, not responding to administration of caffeine. With the continuous recording during administration of the different antiepileptic drugs, the lack of effect could be seen when there was no longer a clinical correlate as the infant was now ventilated.

Posthemorrhagic ventricular dilatation in a late preterm infant

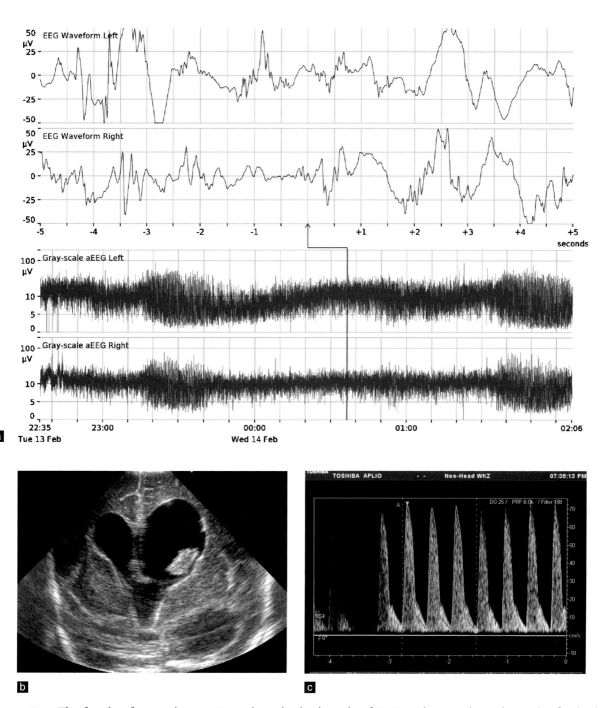

Figure 7.7 This female infant was born at 35 weeks with a birthweight of 2240 g. She was admitted 2 weeks after birth to the NICU for treatment of her posthemorrhagic ventricular dilatation. Her fontanelle was tense on admission with widening of the sutures. Her IVH was presumably of antenatal onset and her first ultrasound scan was performed when she developed a tense fontanelle associated with rapid increase in head circumference.

(a) Cranial ultrasound showed severe ventricular dilatation and associated periventricular cystic leukomalacia. A Doppler ultrasound (b) showed a high systolic peak with a resistance index of 0.93.

(c) aEEG was performed before insertion of the reservoir and showed a normal sleep–wake pattern. The aEEG was repeated after reducing her intracranial pressure and did not show a change in the background pattern.

Preterm infant developing large GMH-IVH

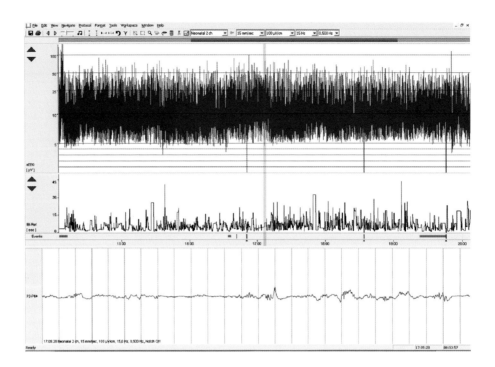

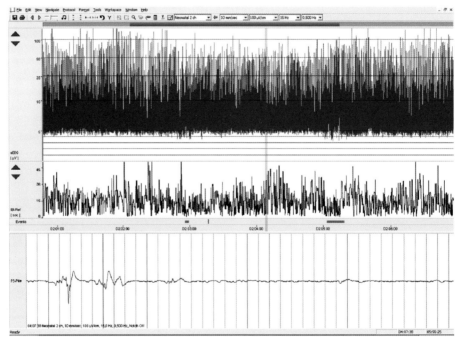

Figure 7.8 This twin was born at 27 gestational weeks and was initially doing well on CPAP. However, on the second day of life a pneumothorax developed which was evacuated. She required surfactant, high-frequency ventilation, and inotrope support. One day later bilateral grade III intraventricular hemorrhages were diagnosed, for which she later required a ventriculo-peritoneal shunt. At 6 months she was suspected of developing cerebral palsy.

The aEEG in (a) was recorded during the first 24 h when she was still on CPAP, and shows a moderately discontinuous background during 6 h with low IBIs. There is no sleep–wake cycling. Panel (b) was recorded after the pneumothorax, in connection with the development of the IVH, and shows a BS pattern with no variability and increased IBIs. No seizures developed. The raised baseline in (b) is probably due to interference from high-frequency ventilation. Also the baseline in (a) looks slightly raised, but the reason for this is not known.

8

Metabolic diseases, brain malformations, and central nervous system infections

This chapter describes examples of aEEG with corresponding EEG traces from newborn infants with various causes of cerebral dysfunction. Infections and hypoglycemia are common in newborn infants, while metabolic diseases and cerebral malformations are rare. Most EEG changes in these conditions are non-specific and include acute stage background abnormalities such as electrocortical background depression and seizures.[15] High bilirubin levels may affect the EEG, mainly with increased slow activity.[156] EEG changes during blood exchange transfusion have also been described.[157] Bilirubin encephalopathy with kernicterus is rare, but can be accompanied by seizures and electrocortical background changes. However, there are no examples including very high bilirubin levels in this Atlas. Specific EEG changes have only been described in a few conditions (see below). The aEEG examples cannot cover all rare conditions but show how the aEEG can be used to give continuous information on brain function and its development during the clinical course in these infants.

Hypoglycemia is probably the most common metabolic cause of acute cerebral dysfunction in newborn infants. Still, there are very few studies evaluating the EEG during hypoglycemic episodes in newborns. Early hypoglycemic EEG changes in adults include an increase in lower EEG frequencies, which is impossible to detect with the aEEG, as shown in full-term infants with moderate hypoglycemia.[158,159] Severe hypoglycemia is associated with aEEG background depression and epileptic seizure activity, as shown in Figure 1.9 in an experimental

settings. Infants with metabolic diseases often develop abundant seizures; urea cycle defects in particular seem to create very intense and long-lasting seizure states.[160]

Burst-suppression EEG background is associated with some severe encephalopathies, such as non-ketotic hyperglycinemia, hemimegalencephaly, and Ohtahara syndrome.[161–164] Other EEG findings, including asymmetries and epileptic seizure activity, may also be present. Some of the background EEG changes associated with these diseases can also be found in the aEEG, as seen in the examples below.

Pyridoxine-dependent seizures are quite rare, but the incidence is probably underestimated.[58] The two examples below of infants with pyridoxine-responsive seizures are probably quite typical in their clinical presentation. They also illustrate the different responses to pyridoxine administration that have been described.[165] Neither of these two infants had the standard EEG pattern, consisting of generalized bursts of 1–4 Hz sharp and slow activity, that has been described as typical for pyridoxine-dependent seizures.[166,167]

Cerebral symptoms due to central nervous system infections or brain malformations are not uncommon. Comparable to metabolic brain dysfunction, the EEG abnormalities are usually non-specific and include background changes and seizures.[168] Changes in the EEG background, such as a multifocal periodic pattern that has been associated with neonatal herpes simplex meningoencephalitis, are not possible to detect with aEEG.[169]

SUMMARY

- Most aEEG/EEG changes due to metabolic diseases, CNS infections, or malformations are non-specific.

- The most common aEEG findings include overall background depression and loss of sleep–wake cycling, and the presence of seizures.

- BS is often present in non-ketotic hyperglycinemia, hemimegalencephaly, and Ohtahara syndrome.

- A standard EEG should be recorded early in all infants with cerebral symptoms due to metabolic disturbances, including hypoglycemia, infections, and cerebral malformations.

Full-term infant with hypoglycemia due to insulinoma

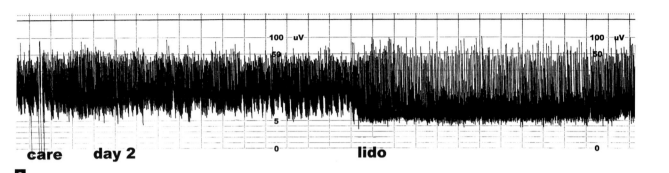

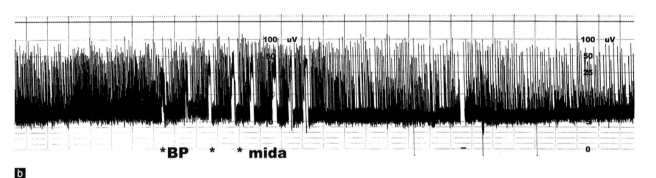

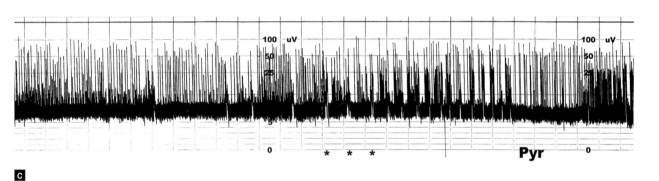

Figure 8.1 This female infant was born at home at 37 weeks' gestation; her birthweight was 3700 g and her Apgar scores were 9 and 10 at 1 and 5 minutes, respectively. Breastfeeding was difficult and the next morning she was found to be hypothermic, sweaty, and pale and was taken to the local hospital, where the first blood glucose was < 0.1 mmol/l. It was difficult to normalize her blood glucose levels and she was intubated and transferred to the regional NICU for further treatment. Her insulin level was increased (15 mIE/l). She was diagnosed to have a gene defect encoding for the protein SUR1 of the pancreatic β cell K_{ATP} channel.

aEEG was initially recorded with an analog machine, started soon after admission, showing suspected repeated ictal discharges on a normal voltage pattern to start with. Following administration of lidocaine, the background pattern became discontinuous with a BS pattern (a). Several hours later she developed clinical (*) as well as subclinical ictal discharges on a BS background. Midazolam was added to the medication and the seizures were temporarily under control (b). In (c) several very small interruptions of the background are seen.

Full-term infant with hypoglycemia due to insulinoma

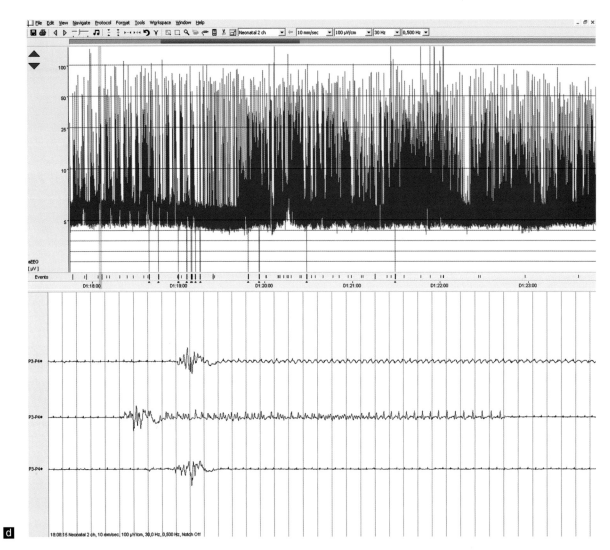

Figure 8.1 *continued* The digital (NicoletOne, Viasys) comparison confirms that these are brief ictal discharges with a very sudden onset and end of the discharge. In (d) a BS is seen without ictal discharges, and (e), recorded on day 4 after birth, shows a certain recovery to a discontinuous background pattern.

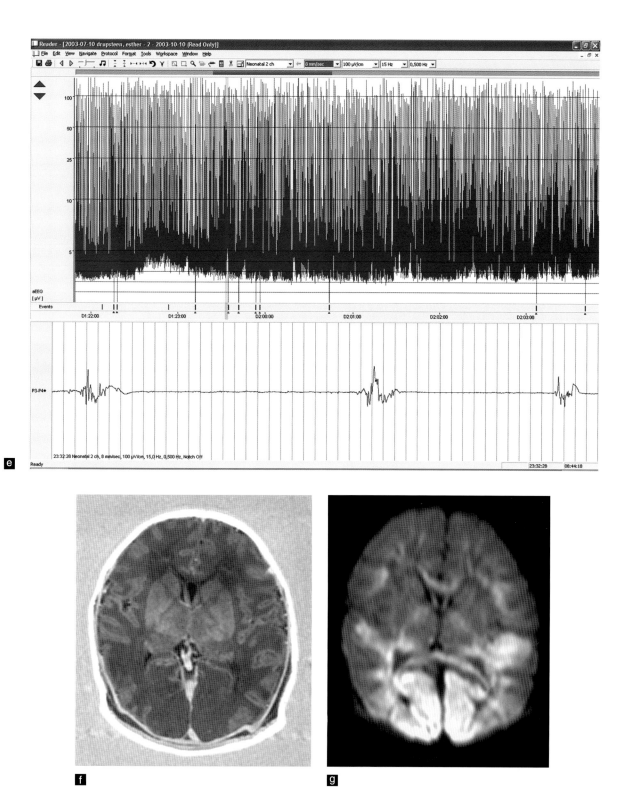

Figure 8.1 *opposite and above* Cranial ultrasound showed extensive increased echogenicity throughout the thalami and the periventricular white matter (not shown). (f and g) MRI performed on day 4 showed extensive injury with loss of gray-white matter differentiation on inversion recovery sequence in the occipital regions and more extensive abnormalities extending anteriorly involving the thalami on diffusion-weighted imaging.

Full-term infant with a long-chain fatty acid disorder

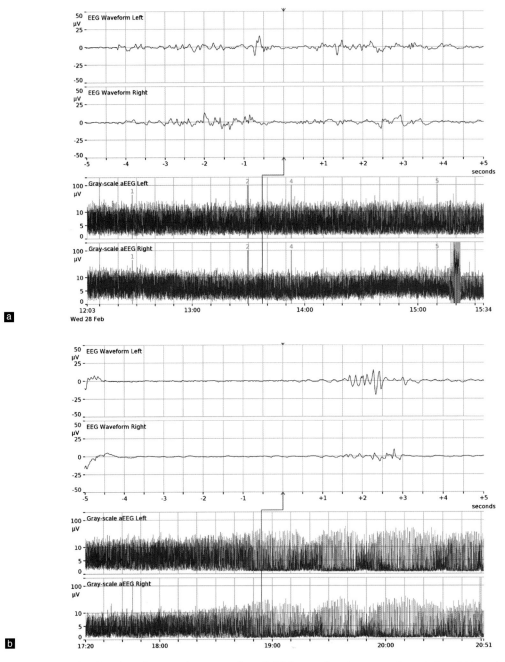

Figure 8.2 This female infant was born as a first child from related parents (cousins) at 35 weeks' gestation with a birth-weight of 2110 g, as the mother had severe pre-eclampsia. The Apgar scores were 4 and 8 at 1 and 5 minutes, respectively. From the beginning she did not feed well and developed rectal bleeding on day 6, which was initially suspected to be due to necrotizing enterocolitis. The blood glucose was normal, but lactate increased to 8 mmol/l. A cardiac ultrasound showed normal ventricular function. Her condition deteriorated 2 days later with desaturations, while on mechanical ventilation, and lactic acidosis (blood lactate 30 mmol/l), and a base excess of – 20 mmol/l. A bowel perforation was suspected and a laparotomy was done. No perforation was found, but her bowel had the appearance of a megacolon and a colostomy was performed. Following surgery she failed to stabilize, with persisting high lactate levels. Cardiac ultrasound was repeated and was now noted to show very poor ventricular contractility. Results from the metabolic screening test suggested a diagnosis of a long-chain hydroxyacyl-CoA-dehydrogenase deficiency several hours later. The final diagnosis was a long chain 3-ketothiolase deficiency. She died in spite of full intensive-care support.

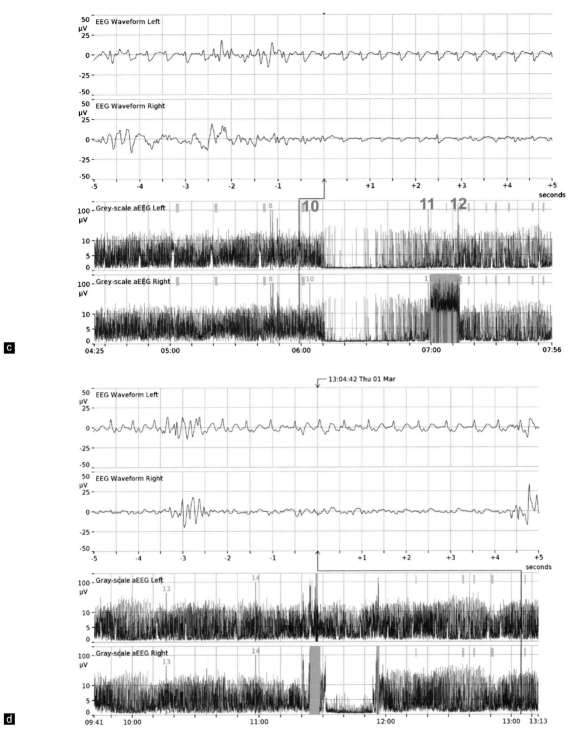

Figure 8.2 *opposite and above* aEEG monitoring was started following surgery and initially showed a moderately discontinuous pattern (a), which spontaneously deteriorated to a sparse BS pattern in (b). Later, left-sided subclinical seizures developed, of duration 2–3 min, interval 15–20 min (c), which are verified by the low-voltage 2 Hz slow and sharp-wave complexes on the left tracing of the original EEG; some rhythmic activity is also present on the right side of this particular seizure. Following administration of phenobarbitone (marker 10, c), the electrocortical background became mainly flat for 25 min, then a sparse BS pattern returned. The raised right-sided aEEG piece of trace, with the red-colored warning between markers 11 and 12, is due to a loose electrode. (d) The nurse reattached the electrode on the right side (red block at 11.30). Following the repositioning of the electrode, a flattening of the recording was seen. The electrodes were found to be too close to each other; following repositioning at a correct interelectrode distance the background pattern was comparable to before the disconnection. Around 20 brief seizures are seen on the left side of the last panel, but no seizures on the right side.

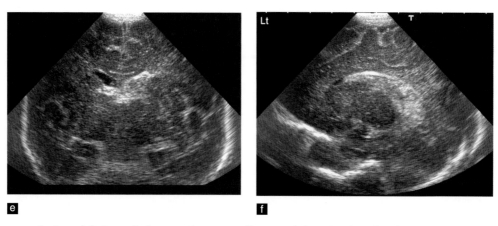

Figure 8.2 *continued*   (e and f) Cranial ultrasound was initially normal, but the day after her surgery a left-sided IVH was noted, with mild left-sided periventricular echogenicity.

Ornithine transcarbamylase (OTC) deficiency

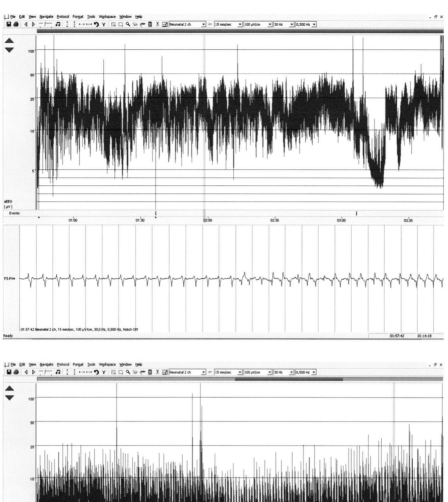

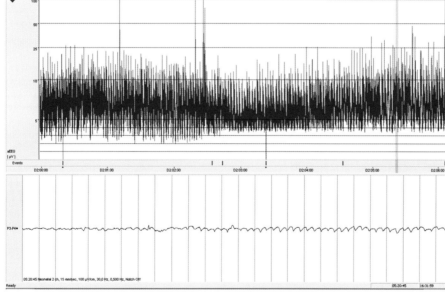

Figure 8.3 This infant was born as the third male child to non-related parents. The pregnancy was normal as was the delivery at 40 weeks' gestational age. Birthweight was 4020 g and Apgar scores were 9 and 10 at 1 and 5 minutes, respectively. When he was 24 h old he started vomiting and became lethargic and tachypneic. Suspected clinical seizures, resembling hiccups, were noted. On arrival at the regional NICU at 4 days of age he was comatose and unresponsive and had severe hyperammonemia (930 µmol/l). Dialysis was initiated within a few hours. The diagnosis of OTC deficiency was later established. He survived the neonatal period but died within some months.

The aEEG was started 3 h after arrival and shows continuously ongoing subclinical status epilepticus (a). At this time-point the infant was very unstable, and needed inotrope support to maintain blood pressure. There is a transient drop in amplitude at time 02:30, but there are no explanatory notes. However, it is possible that this drop could have been caused by hypotension. Panel (b) begins 8 h later, when he was on dialysis, and shows a continuous subclinical status epilepticus.

Non-ketotic hyperglycinemia

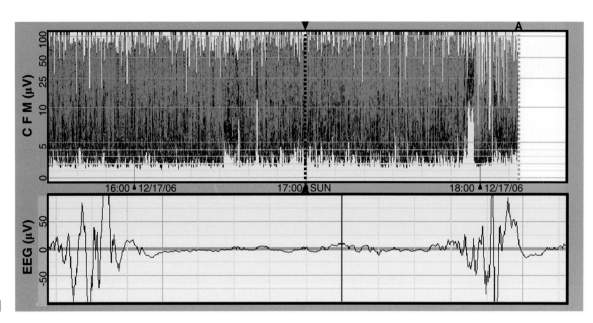

Figure 8.4   This infant was delivered by an elective Cesarean section at 38 weeks and 5 days. He had good Apgar scores, 9 and 10 at 1 and 5 minutes, respectively. His birthweight was 3380 g and his head circumference 35.4 cm. He was noted to be drowsy on day 1, and feeding was poor on day 2, and because of shallow breathing he was admitted to the NICU. He needed mechanical ventilation for 2 weeks. He did not develop clinical seizures. A diagnosis of non-ketotic hyperglycinemia was made. This diagnosis was considered likely on the basis of the clinical history, the dysplastic corpus callosum seen on cranial ultrasound performed after admission and subsequently on MRI, and the BS pattern on the aEEG. The plasma glycine was raised at 2069 μmol/L (the upper limit of normal being 689 μmol/L). The CSF glycine was 309 μmol/L (the upper limit of normal being 8 μmol/L) and the CSF/plasma glycine ratio was 0.15 (normal being 0.07). The urine glycine was 6 times the upper limit of normal.

The aEEG shows a severely discontinuous background pattern (a). Note the almost continuous presence of overload during the bursts. The elevation of the lower margin at 18.00 was not confirmed to be an ictal discharge on the original EEG. (*Courtesy of D Azzopardi and F Cowan.*)

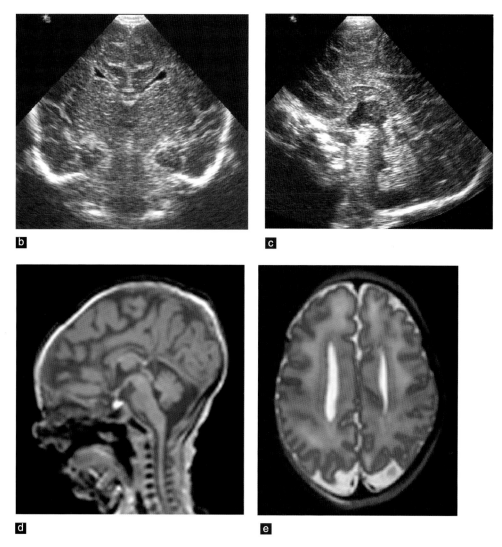

Figure 8.4 *opposite and above*   Cranial ultrasound and MRI showed changes compatible with a dysplastic corpus callosum: the 'bull-horn sign' on the coronal ultrasound (a) view and parallel alignment of the lateral ventricles on the axial MRI (e). The MRI below the ultrasound confirmed the ultrasound findings on the midsagittal view (c, d) and also showed a rather diffuse increased signal intensity of the white matter on the T2 spinecho sequence (e).

Pyridoxine-responsive and pyridoxine-dependent seizures

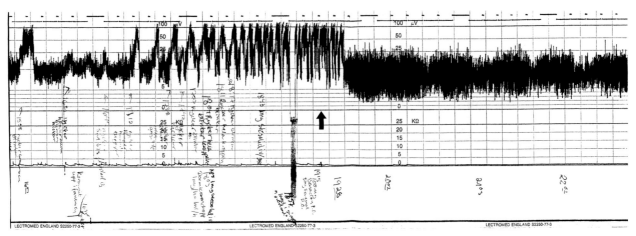

a

Figure 8.5 The two cases shown here illustrate (a) a child with pyridoxine-reponsive seizures, and (b) a child with pyridoxine-dependent seizures. The diagnosis of pyridoxine-dependent seizures is usually made when a child, after an initial response to pyridoxine, develops new seizures when pyridoxine treatment is temporarily discontinued. Since the child in (a) was never challenged, but probably has pyridoxine dependency, the diagnosis is still pyridoxine-responsive seizures.

The figures are shown by permission from reference 165.

(a) This full-term male infant was born after a normal pregnancy, with Apgar scores of 9, 9, and 10 at 1, 5, and 10 min, respectively, an umbilical artery pH of 7.21, and meconium-stained amniotic fluid. He was admitted to the neonatal unit because he was irritable and had moderate metabolic acidosis. Myoclonic seizures started at 12 h and continued for several days in spite of treatment with diazepam, phenobarbitone, lidocaine, and phenytoin. Two standard EEGs showed BS and normal activity, respectively. Seizures recurred later and again antiepileptic treatment with diazepam, phenobarbital, lidocaine, and phenytoin was not effective. This time pyridoxine was given, with immediate effect on the seizure activity (see below). He remained on pyridoxine, and a decision to withdraw the pyridoxine was changed when very subtle episodes of arrested activity occurred with a corresponding left-sided rhythmic theta activity on the EEG. He has a moderate mental retardation.

The aEEG was recorded when the seizures recurred at 15 days. The recurrent electroclinical seizures can be seen as a 'saw-tooth pattern' during the first 4 h of the tracing. The seizures were totally abolished 15 min after 100 mg pyridoxine was given orally (at the arrow) through the nasogastric feeding tube (there was no iv pyridoxine available). After the administration of pyridoxine the aEEG showed continuous background with a slightly periodic pattern (low minimum amplitude but normal maximum voltage) and cyclical fluctuations suggestive of sleep–wake cycling.[165]

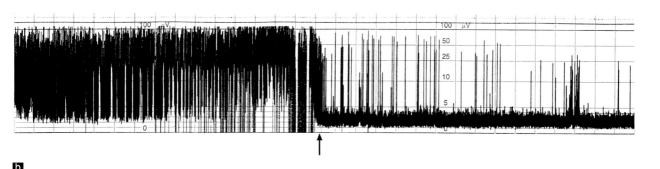

b

Figure 8.5 *opposite and above*   (b) This female infant was born at 34 weeks' gestation with Apgar scores of 6, 8, and 9 at 1, 5, and 10 min, respectively, and a birthweight of 2240 g. The pregnancy was normal except for a routine ultrasound examination at 32 weeks' gestation that showed suspected bowel dilatation. Soon after birth she became restless and irritable. Abdominal ultrasound and X-rays were normal. She had a metabolic acidosis with pH 7.08, base excess −21 mmol/l, and plasma lactate 20 mmol/l. At 12 h she needed sedation (with midazolam and morphine) and mechanical ventilation due to the irritability. On the third day of life she developed multifocal myoclonic seizures. She received iv diazepam and lidocaine with no effect, and was then given 100 mg pyridoxine iv. The seizures stopped within 2 min and she became profoundly hypotonic. A standard EEG on the following day was discontinuous with bilateral epileptiform activity, but the EEG normalized within 3 days. She had no more seizures and was extubated after 5 days. A trial of pyridoxine withdrawal was done when she was 2.5 years old, and resulted in recurrent seizures and continuing pyridoxine medication. Her development is slightly delayed.

The aEEG showed high-amplitude recurrent, almost continuous, electrographic seizure activity concomitant with the clinical seizures. After pyridoxine administration (at the arrow) the aEEG changed dramatically, the electrographic seizure activity ceased almost immediately, and the background amplitude became extremely low in voltage. The aEEG background recovered slowly during the following 8–10 h.

Two infants with Zellweger syndrome

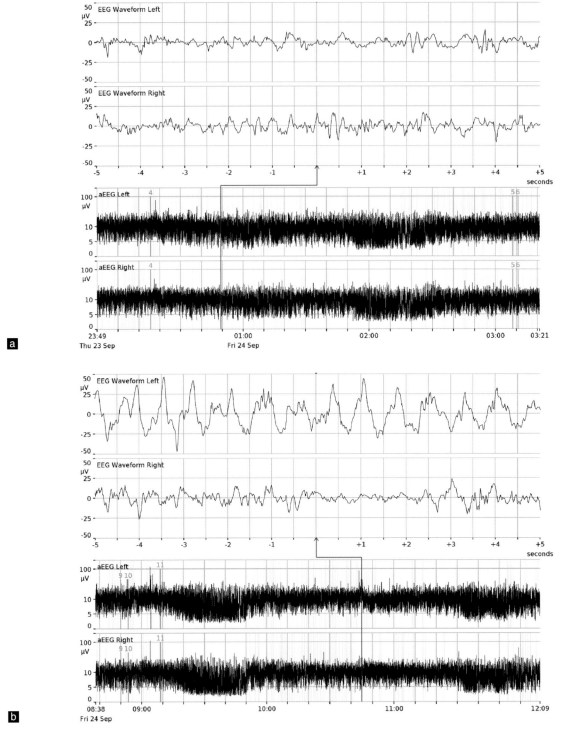

Figure 8.6 (a–d) This male infant was born at 37 weeks with a birthweight of 2830 g. The parents were cousins. Antenatal ultrasound examinations had shown an abnormal posture and length of the lower extremities as well as polyhydramnios. A neuromuscular disorder was suspected. He was born by vaginal delivery and had Apgar scores of 7 and 7 at 1 and 5 minutes, respectively. Following delivery he was noted to be hypotonic and to have a very large anterior and posterior fontanelle. Zellweger syndrome was suspected and subsequently confirmed.

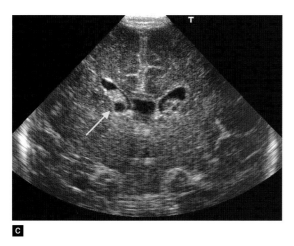
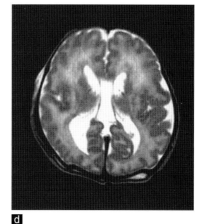

aEEG was started on admission and showed a continuous voltage pattern with some variability. The lower margin of the recording looks rather irregular (a), but there are no ictal discharges present. In panel (b) the sleep–wake pattern is slightly more organized, but the QS periods seems to be more discontinuous than what is normal for his maturity. A very brief electrical discharge, which was entirely subclinical, is seen with sharp and slow-wave complexes of about 1 Hz. There were no more seizures in this trace.

Cranial ultrasound on admission showed typical changes, with bilateral germinolytic cysts and mild ventricular dilatation. Ultrasound of the kidneys showed multiple typical subcortical cysts. Polymicrogyria was suspected with ultrasound, due to the flat appearance of the insula, and confirmed with MRI, as shown on the T2 weighted spin echosequence (d). Reproduced with permission from Leijser LM et al. AJNR 2007; 28:1223–31.

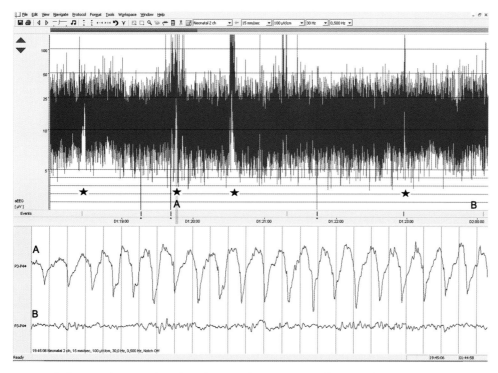

Figure 8.6 *opposite and above* The second male infant was born at 41 weeks' GA after a normal pregnancy and a normal delivery. His birthweight was 3700 g, and Apgar scores were 7, 7, and 7 at 1, 5, and 10 minutes, respectively. However, immediately after birth he was hypotonic with respiratory insufficiency and required intubation 10 min after the delivery. He was noted to have a large anterior fontanelle and wide sutures, a high forehead with a broad nasal ridge, low-set ears, adducted feet, and hypospadia. MRI showed perisylvian polymicrogyria, ventricular dilatation, and pachygyria. Zellweger syndrome was suspected and later confirmed. He died within a few weeks.

The aEEG from his second day of life shows a mainly continuous background without sleep–wake cycling during the 6-h recording (e). Four brief seizures are present in the recording (marked *); at A there is a clinical note 'sleeping'. B shows a representative sample of the EEG background.

Meningitis with group B streptococcus

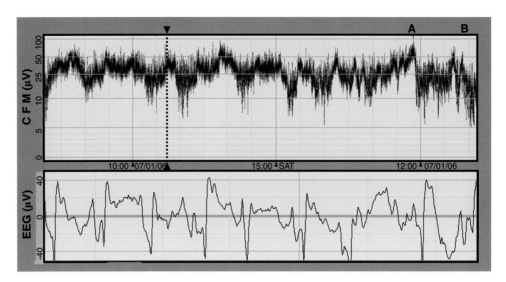

A, clinical seizure; B, care.

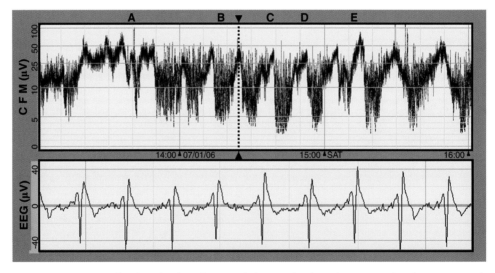

A, phenobarbitone; B, EEG; C, midazolam loading dose; D, lidocaine loading dose; E, midazolam increased.

Figure 8.7 This female infant was born at 35 weeks and was initially doing well. When she was almost 4 weeks old she presented in casualty with grunting. She developed apneic spells shortly after admission and was intubated and ventilated in the NICU. Group B streptococci were present in the blood culture. A lumbar puncture was not performed initially, but in view of the extensive abnormalities seen on neuroimaging it was concluded that she also had group B streptococcus meningitis. Intensive care was eventually withdrawn due to the severe clinical condition.

The initial aEEG showed a mainly subclinical status epilepticus, although she had a clinical seizure at A in (a). Phenobarbitone, midazolam, and lidocaine were administered in (b) without any clear effect on the seizures. All aEEG suspected seizures were confirmed with the original EEG, and seen as sharp and slow-wave complexes of 1 or 1.5 s duration. Her background pattern deteriorated over time to a more discontinuous pattern (not shown). A prolonged single seizure is seen 12 hours later in panel (c).

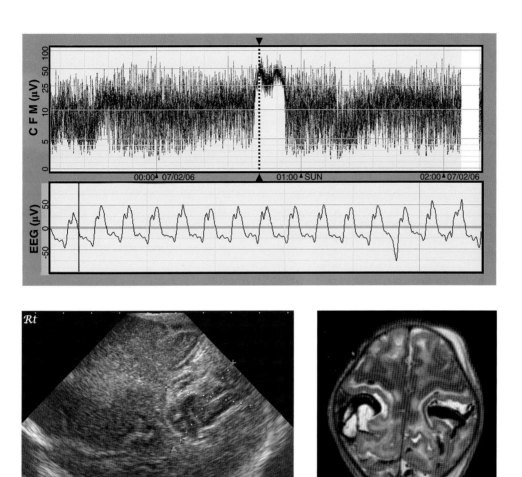

Figure 8.7 *opposite and above* Cranial ultrasound showed areas of increased echogenicity suggestive of hemorrhagic necrosis (d). The parasagittal view showed bilateral areas of mixed echogenicity and echolucency. These lesions were subsequently confirmed on MRI (T2-weighted spin echo sequence) to be areas of hemorrhagic necrosis (e).

Encephalitis with *Bacillus cereus* in a preterm infant

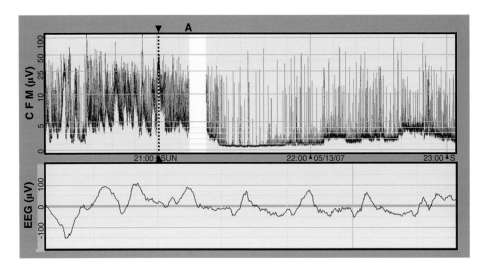

A, phenobarbitone.

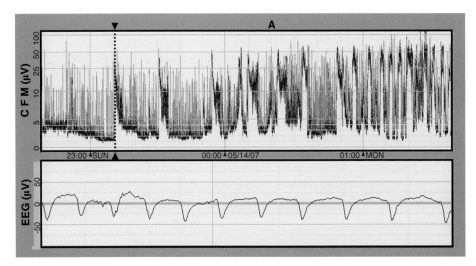

A, lidocaine loading dose.

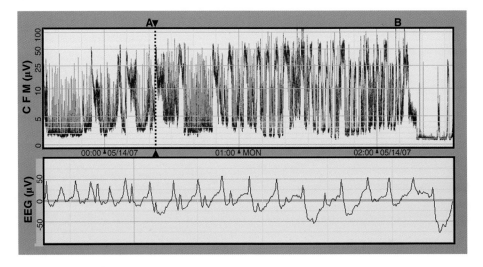

A, lidocaine loading dose; B, clonazepam loading dose.

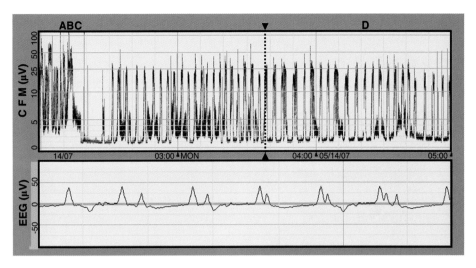

Clonazepam was increased at A, B, C, and D.

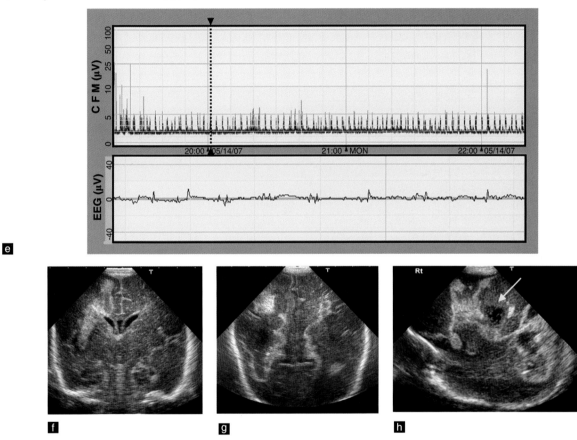

Figure 8.8 *opposite and above* This male infant was born at 31 weeks' gestation, with a birthweight of 1600 g. He was initially doing well but developed a rapidly progressing sepsis and meningoencephalitis with *Bacillus cereus* when he was 60 h old. He died 36 h after the onset of the infection in spite of full intensive-care support.

aEEG was started following the onset of the septicemia and encephalitis. At the onset of the recording a saw-tooth pattern with repetitive seizures can be seen, which was verified by the EEG below (a). Following administration of phenobarbitone (A) the background pattern changes to a very depressed BS pattern, with sparse bursts appearing with intervals of several minutes. (b) There is a recurrence of the seizures and a loading dose of lidocaine is administered without any effect (A). (c) There is a period of status epilepticus. A loading dose of clonazepam is given (B) which stops the status but changes the tracing to an almost inactive recording. (d) A recurrence of the status epilepticus occurs on a flat background and the clonazepam is increased several times without any effect. Panel (e) shows an almost isoelectric recording with some very low-voltage possible ictal discharges.

Cranial ultrasound was normal on admission, but the white matter became severely echogenic (coronal views, f and g) and cystic evolution was seen within the following 12 h (arrow)(h).

Encephalitis with parecho virus

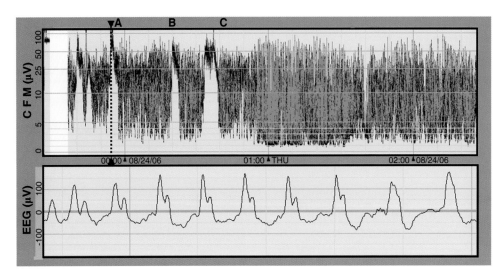

A, seizure; B, central line; C, midazolam

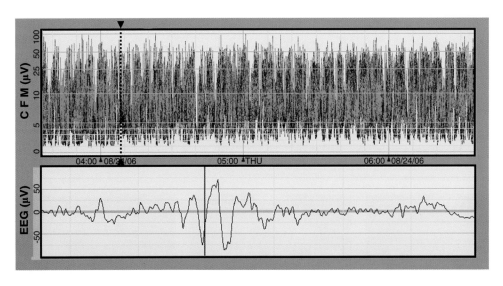

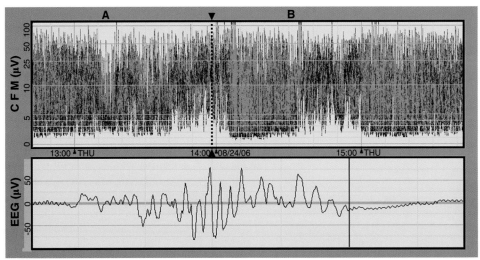

(A–B), standard EEG done, showing multifocal short ictal discharges between 5 and 10 s.

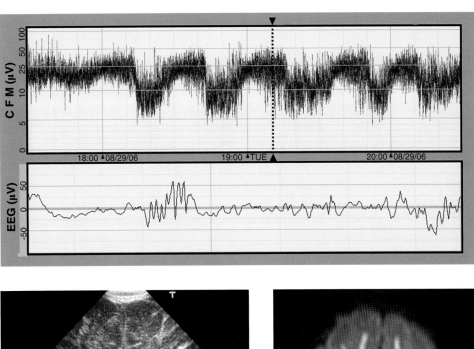

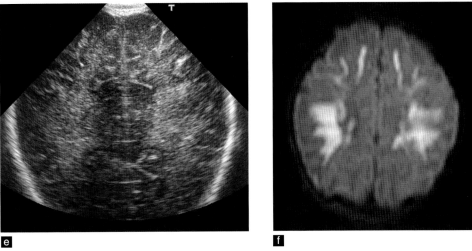

Figure 8.9 *opposite and above*   This female infant was born at 37 gestational weeks. She did well initially but developed fever when she was one week old. The following day she had diarrhea, and later also apneas and hemiconvulsions. A mild diffuse rash was seen over the trunk. Parecho virus was identified in blood and cerebrospinal fluid with polymerase chain reaction (PCR). Her development at 9 months showed a mild delay in milestones but did not suggest the development of cerebral palsy.

The aEEG was started when the clinical seizures developed, and shows five seizures on a slightly discontinuous background, confirmed by the EEG as polymorphic sharp and slow-wave complexes of 1 Hz. A continuous infusion of midazolam was started (C, panel a) with good anticonvulsive effect, rendering the overall electrocortical background more discontinuous. In (b) the lower margin was irregular and this DNV-BS pattern was suspected of containing short ictal discharges. (c) A full standard EEG was therefore made (between A and B) and did indeed confirm multifocal brief ictal discharges lasting between 5 and 10 s. Recovery of the electrocortical background was quite slow. (d) The aEEG five days after admission. The aEEG background is continuous, with a cyclicity resembling a sleep–wake cycling pattern, although the suggested QS periods are briefer and more frequent than what could be expected.

Cranial ultrasound, coronal view angling backwards, performed on admission, showed increased bilateral echogenicity of the periventricular white matter (e). An MRI performed 5 days following onset of seizures showed extensive bilateral DWI changes in the periventricular and deep white matter (f).

Incontinentia pigmenti

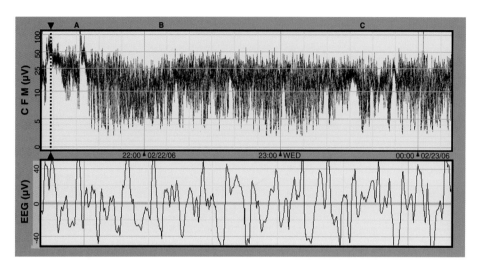

A, midazolam 0.05 mg/kg iv; B, hiccups; C, clinical seizure.

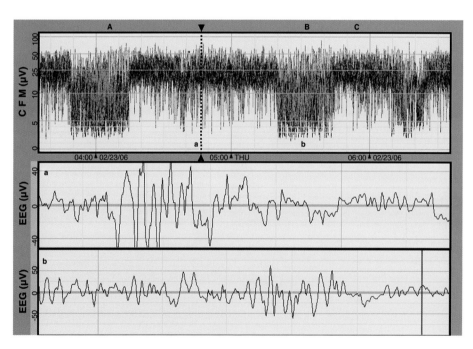

A and B, clinical seizures; C, phenobarbitone.

Figure 8.10 This female infant was born at term with a birthweight of 3945 g. She did well to start with until she developed seizures on day 3. She was extremely irritable, had an exanthema, and she was initially suspected of a viral encephalitis. Her skin lesions were, however, rather localized on her legs and arms and the pediatric dermatologist performed a skin biopsy as incontinentia pigmenti was suspected and subsequently confirmed. The illustration (c) shows her linear skin lesions at 6 weeks of age. Her development was abnormal, with the development of epilepsy when she was 8 months old. The epilepsy was difficult to control.

aEEG was started immediately following admission, as she had a clinical seizure. Two ictal discharges are seen at the start of the recording and several more are present in (a), which resembles a saw-tooth pattern. The ictal discharges were confirmed by the original EEG, in the figure from the first seizure with sharp and slow-wave complexes of less than 1 Hz. (b) A very unusual and abnormal background pattern is seen; periods with continuous activity but with no variability are intermixed with abrupt onset of periods of a more discontinuous pattern. No clear ictal discharges were seen on the original EEG either during the periods of depression or during more continuous activity.

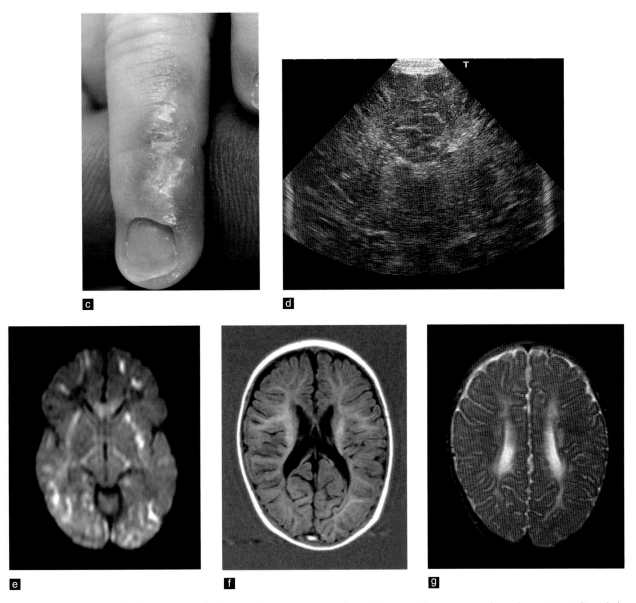

Figure 8.10 *opposite and above*   Cranial ultrasound on admission showed increased periventricular echogenicity (d) and the MRI performed 3 days after admission showed rather extensive signal intensity changes best seen with DWI (e). A repeat MRI performed at 9 months shows loss of white matter and a delay in myelination (inversion image, f) and early signs of gliotic white matter damage (T2 spin echo sequence, g).

Hemimegalencephaly

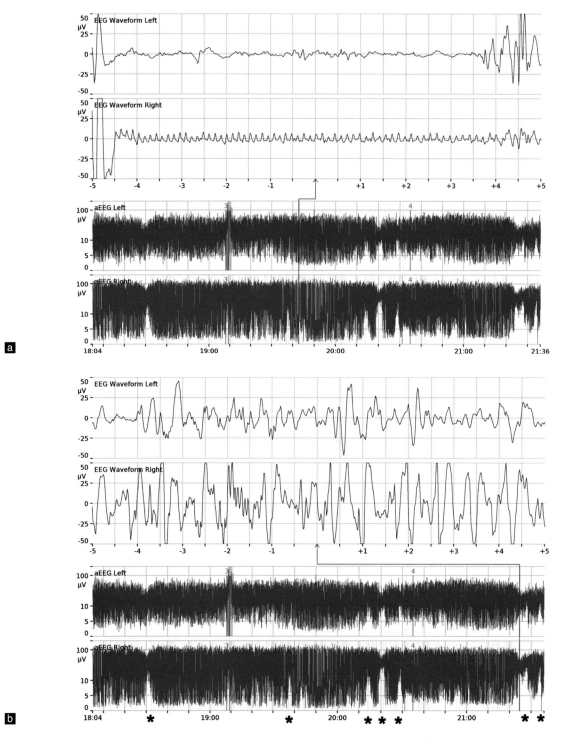

Figure 8.11   This male infant was born at 38 weeks' gestation with a birthweight of 3740 g. Apgar scores were 9 and 10 at 1 and 5 min, respectively. A linear nevus sebaceous was seen over the nose (c), and he developed clinical seizures within an hour after delivery. Ultrasound and later MRI showed changes of the right hemisphere suggestive of hemimegalencephaly. He was diagnosed with Jadassohn syndrome, which includes partial seizures or infantile spasms, mental retardation, hemi-macrocrania, and ocular abnormalities. His seizures were difficult to control and a hemispherectomy was done when he was 2 years old. His development is severely delayed.

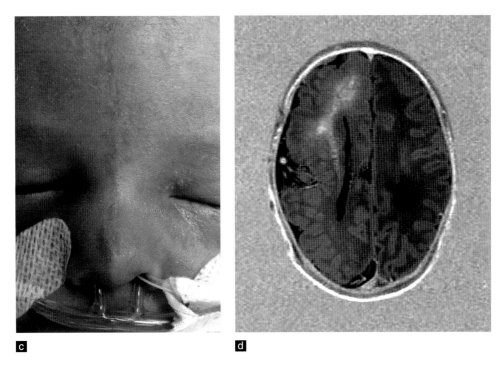

Figure 8.11 *opposite and above* aEEG showed an asymmetry in the background pattern, with more discontinuous and high-voltage amplitude on the right affected side and several ictal discharges mainly on the right side (*) (panel a and b).

MRI, T1-weighted sequence (inversion recovery (d)), shows an enlarged right hemisphere with extensive cortical dysplasia. The increased signal intensity adjacent to the right ventricle was due to calcification which was confirmed on CT (not shown).

Tuberous sclerosis

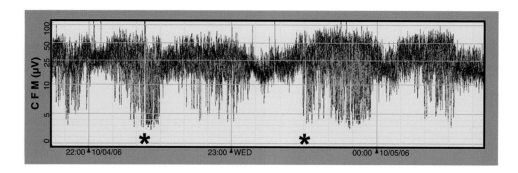

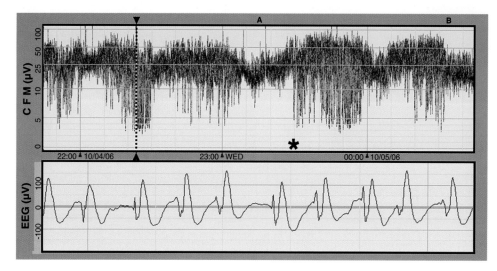

A, Care; B, lipsmacking.

Figure 8.12 This male infant was born at 40 weeks' gestation, with a birthweight of 3660 g. His Apgar scores were 9 and 10 at 1 and 5 mins, respectively. When he was 2 days old, he developed right-sided hemiconvulsions and was admitted to the NICU. A cardiac ultrasound showed a single rhabdomyoma, and the diagnosis of tuberous sclerosis was suspected. His seizures were never completely controlled and, following several periods of status epilepticus, a left hemispherectomy was eventually performed when he was 6 months old.

The aEEG background was mainly continuous, but had an appearance resembling sleep–wake cycling, although the discontinuous periods did not look typical for QS periods in a full-term infant (arrows). The real EEG showed that these changes were due to brief ictal discharges (sharp–slow-wave complexes of about 1 s duration) lasting about 10 s. As the marker line completely obscures the ictal discharge the same panel is shown twice.

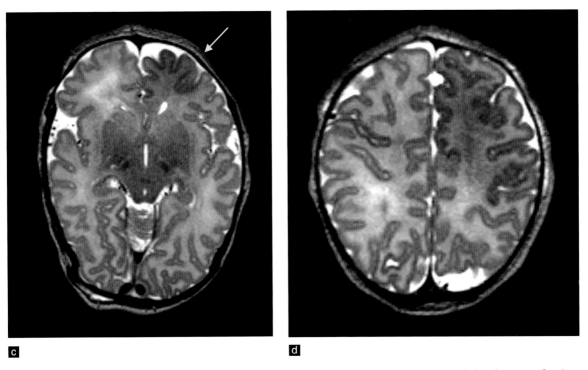

Figure 8.12 *opposite and above*   Cranial ultrasound did not show any clear abnormalities, and the diagnosis focal cortical dysplasia was made with MRI (T2 spin echo sequence) (c (arrow) and d).

Ohtahara syndrome

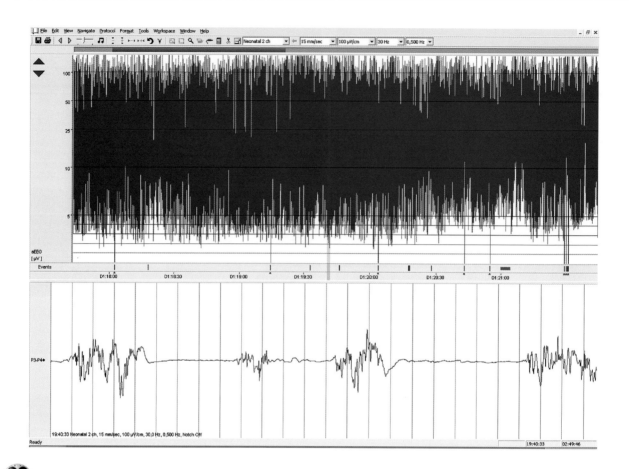

Figure 8.13 This girl was the third child of healthy non-related parents. The pregnancy and delivery at 38 weeks' gestation were normal. Birthweight was 3610 g and Apgar scores were 9, 10, and 10, at 1, 5, and 10 minutes, respectively. She was initially doing well but was readmitted to the hospital at 6 days due to lethargy and feeding problems, with a weight loss > 10%. Brief suspected clonic seizures were noted 3–4 times per day. Repeated initial EEGs showed BS but no seizures. An extensive neurometabolic investigation was performed, but did not give a specific diagnosis. From one month of age an increasing number of myoclonic seizures developed, sometimes accompanied by apnea. She received antiepileptic treatment, including corticosteroids and pyridoxine, without improvement of the seizures, and she died at 3 months of age. The clinical picture together with the continuing BS on EEG led to the diagnosis of Ohtahara syndrome.

The neonatal MRI was considered to be normal. The 4-h aEEG was recorded on postnatal day 10 and shows BS but no seizures.

(*Courtesy of Katarina Strand-Brodd*).

Intracranial tumor (teratoma)

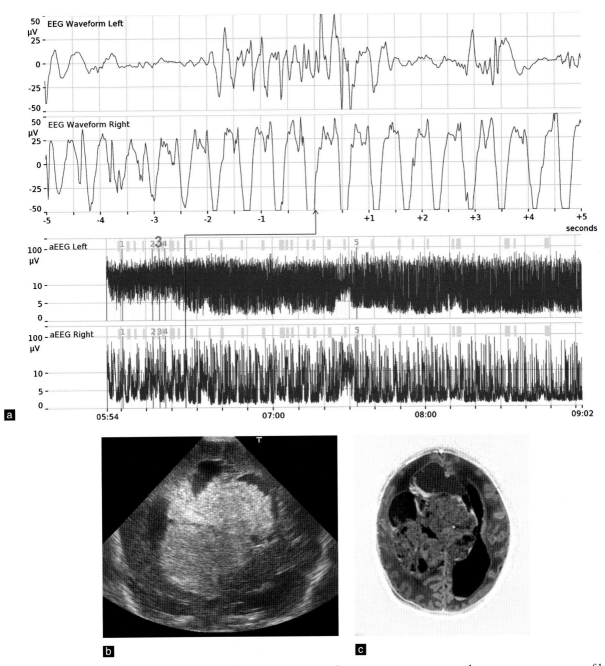

Figure 8.14   This female infant was born at 36 weeks' gestation, by ventouse extraction as there was poor progress of labor. The Apgar scores were 6 and 9 at 1 and 5 minutes, respectively. Her birth weight was 3000 g (+1 SD), length 51 cm (+2 SD), head circumference 37 cm (>>+2½ SD). She developed seizures within some hours after delivery and was referred to the NICU. She died 2 weeks later.

aEEG was started soon after admission and showed a unilateral status epilepticus of the affected right hemisphere (a). The left hemisphere, which is under pressure, starts with a continuous voltage pattern and changes to a more discontinuous voltage pattern following administration of a loading dose of phenobarbitone at marker 3. The discharges do not resolve completely but are less frequent and less prominent and mainly right-sided, although the seizure detection (orange blocks) continues to detect discharges from both hemispheres.

Cranial ultrasound on admission showed a large echogenic mass with an irregular outline, mainly seen in the right hemisphere (b). An MRI (inversion recover sequence) confirmed the finding of a brain tumor, a suspected teratoma (c). Surgery was not performed; postmortem histology confirmed the diagnosis of a teratoma.

References

1. Steriade M, Gloor P, Llinás RR, Lopes da. Report of IFCN Committee on basic mechanisms. Basic mechanisms of cerebral rhythmic activities. Electroencephalogr Clin Neurophysiol 1990; 76: 481–508.

2. Kostovic I, Jovanov-Milosevic N. The development of cerebral connections during the first 20–45 weeks' gestation. Semin Fetal Neonatal Med 2006; 11: 415–22.

3. Vanhatalo S, Kaila K. Development of neonatal EEG activity: from phenomenology to physiology. Semin Fetal Neonatal Med 2006; 11: 471–8.

4. Vanhatalo S, Voipio J, Kaila K. Full-band EEG (fbEEG): a new standard for clinical electroencephalography. Clin EEG Neurosci 2005; 36: 311–17.

5. Vanhatalo S, Tallgren P, Andersson S et al. DC-EEG discloses prominent, very slow wave activity patterns during sleep in preterm infants. Clin Neurophysiol 2002; 113: 1822–5.

6. Maynard DE. EEG analysis using an analogue frequency analyser and a digital computer. Electroencephalogr Clin Neurophysiol 1967; 23: 487.

7. Maynard D, Prior PF, Scott DF. Device for continuous monitoring of cerebral activity in resuscitated patients. Br Med J 1969; 4: 545–6.

8. Prior PF. EEF monitoring and evoked potentials in brain ischaemia. Br J Anaesth 1985; 57: 63–81.

9. Prior PF, Maynard DE. Monitoring cerebral function. Long-term recordings of cerebral electrical activity and evoked potentials. Amsterdam: Elsevier, 1986: 1–441.

10. Rosén I. The physiological basis for continuous electroencephalogram monitoring in the neonate. Clin Perinatol 2006; 33: 593–611.

11. Viniker DA, Maynard DE, Scott DF. Cerebral function monitor studies in neonates. Clin Electroenceph 1984; 15: 185–92.

12. Bjerre I, Hellström-Westas L, Rosén I, Svenningsen NW. Monitoring of cerebral function after severe birth asphyxia in infancy. Arch Dis Child 1983; 58: 997–1002.

13. Verma UL, Archbald F, Tejani N, Handwerker SM. Cerebral function monitor in the neonate. I. Normal patterns. Dev Med Child Neurol 1984; 26: 154–61.

14. Archbald F, Verma UL, Tejani NA, Handwerker SM. Cerebral function monitor in the neonate. II. Birth asphyxia. Dev Med Child Neurol 1984; 26: 162–8.

15. Watanabe K, Hayakawa F, Okumura A. Neonatal EEG: a powerful tool in the assessment of brain damage in preterm infants. Brain Dev 1999; 21: 361–72.

16. Agardh CD, Rosén I. Neurophysiological recovery after hypoglycemic coma in the rat: correlation with cerebral metabolism. J Cereb Blood Flow Metab 1983; 3: 78–85.

17. Inder TE, Buckland L, Williams CE et al. Lowered electroencephalographic spectral edge frequency predicts the presence of cerebral white matter injury in premature infants. Pediatrics 2003; 111: 27–33.

18. Jasper HH. The ten-twenty electrode system of the International Federation. Electroencephalogr Clin Neurophysiol 1958; 10: 371–3.

19. Jasper HH. The ten-twenty electrode system of the International Federation. In: International Federation of Societies for Electroencephalography and Clinical Neurophysiology. Recommendations for the practice

of clinical electroencephalography. Amsterdam: Elsevier, 1983: 3–10.

20. Dreyfus-Brisac C. Neonatal electroencephalography. In: Scarpelli EM, Cosmi V, eds. Reviews of Perinatal Medicine. New York: Raven Press, 1979: 379–485.

21. Torres F, Anderson C. The normal EEG of the human newborn. J Clin Neurophysiol 1985; 2: 89–103.

22. Lombroso CT. Neonatal polygraphy in full-term and premature infants: a review of normal and abnormal findings. J Clin Neurophysiol 1985; 2: 105–55.

23. Tharp BR, Scher MS, Clancy RR. Serial EEGs in normal and abnormal infants with birthweights less than 1200 grams – a prospective study with long term follow-up. Neuropediatrics 1989; 20: 64–72.

24. Lamblin MD, Andre M, Challamel MJ et al. Electroencephalography of the premature and term newborn. Maturational aspects and glossary. Neurophysiol Clin 1999; 29: 123–219.

25. Mizrahi EM, Hrachovy RA, Kellaway P. Atlas of Neonatal Encephalography, 3rd edn. Lippincott Williams & Wilkins, Philadelphia: 2004, pp 1–250.

26. Vecchierini M-F, d'Allest A-M, Verpillat P. EEG patterns in 10 extreme premature neonates with normal neurological outcome: qualitative and quantitative data. Brain Dev 2003; 25: 330–7.

27. Connell JA, Oozeer R, Dubowitz V. Continuous 4-channel EEG monitoring: a guide to interpretation, with normal values, in preterm infants. Neuropediatrics 1987; 18: 138–45.

28. Hayakawa M, Okumura A, Hayakawa F et al. Background electroencephalographic (EEG) activities of very preterm infants born at less than 27 weeks gestation: a study on the degree of continuity. Arch Dis Child Fetal Neonatal Ed 2001; 84: F163–7.

29. Hahn JS, Monyer H, Tharp BR. Interburst interval measurements in the EEGs of premature infants with normal neurological outcome. Electroencephalogr Clin Neurophysiol 1989; 73: 410–18.

30. Selton D, Andre M, Hascoet JM. Normal EEG in very premature infants: reference criteria. Clin Neurophysiol 2000; 111: 2116–24.

31. Biagioni E, Frisone MF, Laroche S et al. Maturation of cerebral electrical activity and development of cortical folding in young very preterm infants. Clin Neurophysiol 2007; 118: 53–9.

32. Wikström S, Ley D, Hansen-Pupp I, Rosén I, Hellström-Westas L. Early amplitude integrated EEG correlates with perinatal inflammation and outcome at 2 years in very preterm infants. Submitted

33. Olischar M, Klebermass K, Kuhle S et al. Reference values for amplitude-integrated electroencephalographic activity in preterm infants younger than 30 weeks' gestational age. Pediatrics 2004; 113: e61–6.

34. Greisen G, Hellström-Westas L, Lou H, Rosén I, Svenningsen NW. EEG depression and germinal layer haemorrhage in the new-born. Acta Paediatr Scand 1987; 76: 519–25.

35. Victor S, Appleton RE, Beirne M, Marson AG, Weindling AM. Spectral analysis of electroencephalography in premature newborn infants: normal ranges. Pediatr Res 2005; 57: 336–41.

36. West CR, Harding JE, Williams CE, Gunning MI, Battin MR. Quantitative electroencephalographic patterns in normal preterm infants over the first week after birth. Early Hum Dev 2006; 82: 43–51.

37. Hellström-Westas L, Rosén I, Svenningsen NW. Cerebral function monitoring in extremely small low birthweight (ESLBW) infants during the first week of life. Neuropediatrics 1991; 22: 27–32.

38. Kuhle S, Klebermass K, Olischar M et al. Sleep–wake cycling in preterm infants below 30 weeks of gestational age. Preliminary results of a prospective amplitude-integrated EEG study. Wien Klin Wochenschr 2001; 113: 219–23.

39. Thornberg E, Thiringer K. Normal patterns of cerebral function monitor traces in term and preterm neonates. Acta Paediatr Scand 1990; 79: 20–5.

40. Sisman J, Campbell DE, Brion LP. Amplitude-integrated EEG in preterm infants: maturation of background pattern and amplitude voltage with postmenstrual age and gestational age. J Perinatol 2005; 25: 391–6.

41. Burdjalov VF, Baumgart S, Spitzer AR. Cerebral function monitoring: a new scoring system for the evaluation of brain maturation in neonates. Pediatrics 2003; 112: 855–61.

42. al Naqeeb N, Edwards AD, Cowan FM, Azzopardi D. Assessment of neonatal encephalopathy by amplitude-integrated electroencephalography. Pediatrics 1999; 103: 1263–71.

43. Gluckman PD, Wyatt JS, Azzopardi D et al. Selective head cooling with mild systemic hypothermia after neonatal encephalopathy: multicentre randomised trial. Lancet 2005; 365: 663–70.

44. Hellström-Westas L, Rosén I, de Vries LS, Greisen G. Amplitude integrated EEG: classification and interpretation in preterm and term infants. Neoreviews 2006; 7: e76–87.

45. Hellström-Westas L, Westgren U, Rosén I, Svenningsen NW. Lidocaine treatment of severe

seizures in newborn infants. I. Clinical effects and cerebral electrical activity monitoring. Acta Paediatr Scand 1988; 77: 79–84.

46. Bell AH, Greisen G, Pryds O. Comparison of the effects of phenobarbitone and morphine administration on EEG activity in preterm babies. Acta Paediatr 1993; 82: 35–9.

47. Young GB, da Silva OP. Effects of morphine on the electroencephalograms of neonates: a prospective, observational study. Clin Neurophysiol 2000; 111: 1955–60.

48. Nguyen The Tich S, Vecchierini MF, Debillon T, Pereon Y. Effects of sufentanil on electroencephalogram in very and extremely preterm neonates. Pediatrics 2003; 111: 123–8.

49. van Leuven K, Groenendaal F, Toet MC et al. Midazolam and amplitude integrated EEG in asphyxiated full-term neonates. Acta Paediatr 2004; 93: 1221–7.

50. Hellström-Westas L, Klette H, Thorngren-Jerneck K, Rosén I. Early prediction of outcome with aEEG in preterm infants with large intraventricular hemorrhages. Neuropediatrics 2001; 32: 319–24.

51. Hellström-Westas L, Bell AH, Skov L, Greisen G, Svenningsen NW. Cerebroelectrical depression following surfactant treatment in preterm neonates. Pediatrics 1992; 89: 643–7.

52. Eaton DG, Wertheim D, Oozeer R, Dubowitz LM, Dubowitz V. Reversible changes in cerebral activity associated with acidosis in preterm neonates. Acta Paediatr 1994; 83: 486–92.

53. West CR, Groves AM, Williams CE et al. Early low cardiac output is associated with compromised electroencephalographic activity in very preterm infants. Pediatr Res 2006; 59: 610–15.

54. Victor S, Marson AG, Appleton RE, Beirne M, Weindling AM. Relationship between blood pressure, cerebral electrical activity, cerebral fractional oxygen extraction, and peripheral blood flow in very low birth weight newborn infants. Pediatr Res 2006; 59: 314–19.

55. Victor S, Appleton RE, Beirne M, Marson AG, Weindling AM. Effect of carbon dioxide on background cerebral electrical activity and fractional oxygen extraction in very low birth weight infants just after birth. Pediatr Res 2005; 58: 579–85.

56. Holsti L, Grunau RE, Oberlander TF, Whitfied MF. Prior pain induces heightened motor responses during clustered care in preterm infants in the NICU. Early Hum Dev 2005; 81: 293–302.

57. Hellström-Westas L, de Vries LS, Rosén I. An Atlas of Amplitude-Integrated EEGs in the Newborn. London: Parthenon Publishing, 2003, pp 1–150.

58. Baxter P. Epidemiology of pyridoxine dependent and pyridoxine responsive seizures in the UK. Arch Dis Child 1999; 81: 431–3.

59. Sheth RD, Hobbs GR, Mullett M. Neonatal seizures: incidence, onset, and etiology by gestational age. J Perinatol 1999; 19: 40–3.

60. Tharp BR. Neonatal seizures and syndromes. Epilepsia 2002; 43 (Suppl 3): 2–10.

61. Tekgul H, Gauvreau K, Soul J et al. The current etiologic profile and neurodevelopmental outcome of seizures in term newborn infants. Pediatrics 2006; 117: 1270–80.

62. Sheth RD. Electroencephalogram confirmatory rate in neonatal seizures. Pediatr Neurol 1999; 20: 27–30.

63. Ronen GM, Penney S, Andrews W. The epidemiology of clinical neonatal seizures in Newfoundland: a population-based study. J Pediatr 1999; 134: 71–5.

64. Saliba RM, Annegers JF, Waller DK, Tyson JE, Mizrahi EM. Incidence of neonatal seizures in Harris County, Texas, 1992–1994. Am J Epidemiol 1999; 150: 763–9.

65. Hellström-Westas L, Blennow G, Lindroth M, Rosén I, Svenningsen NW. Low risk of seizure recurrence after early withdrawal of antiepileptic treatment in the neonatal period. Arch Dis Child 1995; 72: F97–101.

66. Connell J, Oozeer R, de Vries L, Dubowitz V. Continuous EEG monitoring of neonatal seizures: diagnostic and prognostic considerations. Arch Dis Child 1989; 64: 452–8.

67. Helmers SL, Constantinou JE, Newburger JW et al. Perioperative electroencephalographic seizures in infants undergoing repair of complex congenital cardiac defects. Electroencephalogr Clin Neurophysiol 1997; 102: 27–36.

68. Connell J, de Vries L, Oozeer R et al. Predictive value of early continuous electroencephalogram monitoring in ventilated preterm infants with intraventricular hemorrhage. Pediatrics 1988; 82: 337–43.

69. Laroia N, Guillet R, Burchfiel J, McBride MC. EEG background as predictor of electrographic seizures in high-risk neonates. Epilepsia 1998; 39: 545–51.

70. Murray DM, Ryan CA, Boylan GB, Fitzgerald AP, Connolly S. Prediction of seizures in asphyxiated neonates: correlation with continuous video-electroencephalographic monitoring. Pediatrics 2006; 118: 41–6.

71. Hellström-Westas L, Rosén I, Svenningsen NW. Silent seizures in sick infants in early life. Acta Paediatr Scand 1985; 74: 741–8.

72. Clancy RR, Legido A, Lewis D. Occult neonatal seizures. Epilepsia 1988; 29: 256–61.

73. Mizrahi EM, Kellaway P. Characterization and classification of neonatal seizures. Neurology 1987; 37: 1837–44.

74. Volpe JJ. Neurology of the Newborn, 4th edn. WB Saunders Company: Philadelphia, PA, 2000: 178–214.

75. Scher MS, Aso K, Beggarly ME et al. Electrographic seizures in preterm and full-term neonates: clinical correlates, associated brain lesions, and risk for neurologic sequelae. Pediatrics 1993; 91: 128–34.

76. Scher MS, Alvin J, Gaus L, Minnigh B, Painter MJ. Uncoupling of EEG-clinical neonatal seizures after antiepileptic drug use. Pediatr Neurol 2003; 28: 277–80.

77. Murray DM, Boylan GB, Ali I et al. Defining the gap between electrographic seizure burden, clinical expression, and staff recognition of neonatal seizures. Arch Dis Child Fetal Neonatal Ed 2008 (in press); published online 11 July 2007.

78. Radvanyi-Bouvet MF, Vallecalle MH, Morel-Kahn F, Relier JP, Dreyfus-Brisac C. Seizures and electrical discharges in premature infants. Neuropediatrics 1985; 16: 143–8.

79. Connell J, Oozeer R, de Vries L, Dubowitz LM, Dubowitz V. Clinical and EEG response to anticonvulsants in neonatal seizures. Arch Dis Child 1989; 64: 459–64.

80. Toet MC, van der Meij W, de Vries LS, Uiterwaal CSPM, van Huffelen AC. Comparison between simultaneously recorded amplitude integrated EEG (cerebral function monitor (CFM)) and standard EEG in neonates. Pediatrics 2002; 109: 772–9.

81. Boylan GB, Rennie JM, Pressler RM et al. Phenobarbitone, neonatal seizures, and video-EEG. Arch Dis Child Fetal Neonatal Ed 2002; 86: F165–70.

82. Oliveira AJ, Nunes ML, Haertel LM, Reis FM, da Costa JC. Duration of rhythmic EEG patterns in neonates: new evidence for clinical and prognostic significance of brief rhythmic discharges. Clin Neurophysiol 2000; 111: 1646–53.

83. Clancy RR, Legido A. The exact ictal and interictal duration of electroencephalographic neonatal seizures. Epilepsia 1987; 28: 537–41.

84. Scher MS, Hamid MY, Steppe DA, Beggarly ME, Painter MJ. Ictal and interictal electrographic seizure

durations in preterm and term neonates. Epilepsia 1993; 34: 284–8.

85. van Rooij LGM, de Vries LS, Handryastuti S et al. Neurodevelopmental outcome in full term infants with status epilepticus detected with amplitude-integrated electroencephalography. Pediatrics 2007; 120: e354–63.

86. Patrizi S, Holmes GL, Orzalesi M, Allemand F. Neonatal seizures: characteristics of EEG ictal activity in preterm and fullterm infants. Brain Dev 2003; 25: 427–37.

87. Bye AM, Flanagan D. Spatial and temporal characteristics of neonatal seizures. Epilepsia 1995; 36: 1009–16.

88. Tekgul H, Bourgeois BF, Gauvreau K, Bergin AM. Electroencephalography in neonatal seizures: comparison of a reduced and a full 10/20 montage. Pediatr Neurol 2005; 32: 155–61.

89. Shellhaas RA, Saoita AI, Clancy RR. Sensitivity of amplitude-integrated electroencephalography for neonatal seizure detection. Pediatrics 2007; 120: 770–7.

90. Hellström-Westas L. Comparison between tape-recorded and amplitude-integrated EEG monitoring in sick newborn infants. Acta Paediatr 1992; 81: 812–19.

91. Shah DK, MacKay MT, Lavery S et al. The accuracy of bedside EEG monitoring as compared with simultaneous continuous conventional EEG for seizure detection in term infants. Pediatrics 2008 (in press).

92. Van Rooij LG, Toet MC, de Vries LS. Comparison of 2-channel and 1-channel amplitude integrated EEG with respect to seizure-activity and background pattern. (abstract) E-PAS2007: 618446.6.

93. Bennet L, Dean JM, Wassink G, Gunn AJ. Differential effects of hypothermia on early and late epileptiform events after severe hypoxia in preterm fetal sheep. J Neurophysiol 2007; 97: 572–8.

94. Gotman J, Flanagan D, Zhang J, Rosenblatt B. Automatic seizure detection in the newborn: methods and initial evaluation. Electroencephalogr Clin Neurophysiol 1997; 103: 356–62.

95. Navakatikyan MA, Colditz PB, Burke CJ et al. Seizure detection algorithm for neonates based on wave-sequence analysis. Clin Neurophysiol 2006; 117: 1190–203.

96. Lommen CM, Pasman JW, van Kranen VH et al. An algorithm for the automatic detection of seizures in neonatal amplitude-integrated EEG. Acta Paediatr 2007; 96: 674–80.

97. Toet MC, Groenendaal F, Osredkar D, van Huffelen AC, de Vries L. Postneonatal epilepsy

following amplitude-integrated EEG-detected neo-natal seizures. Pediatr Neurol 2005; 32: 241–7.

98. Guillet R, Kwon J. Seizure recurrence and developmental disabilities after neonatal seizures: outcomes are unrelated to use of phenobarbital prophylaxis. J Child Neurol 2007; 22: 389–95.

99. Rowe JC, Holmes GL, Hafford J et al. Prognostic value of the electroencephalogram in term and preterm infants following neonatal seizures. Electroencephalogr Clin Neurophysiol 1985; 60: 183–96.

100. Lombroso CT, Holmes GL. Value of the EEG in neonatal seizures. J Epilepsy 1993; 6: 39–70.

101. McBride MC, Laroia N, Guillet R. Electrographic seizures in neonates correlate with poor neurodevelopmental outcome. Neurology 2000; 55: 506–13.

102. Roberton NRC. Effect of acute hypoxia on blood pressure and electroencephalogram of newborn babies. Arch Dis Child 1969; 44: 719–25.

103. Bunt JE, Gavilanes AW, Reulen JP, Blanco CE, Vles JS. The influence of acute hypoxemia and hypovolemic hypotension on neuronal brain activity measured by the cerebral function monitor in new-born piglets. Neuropediatrics 1996; 27: 260–4.

104. Williams CE, Gunn AJ, Mallard C, Gluckman PD. Outcome after ischemia in the developing brain: an electroencephalographic and histological study. Ann Neurol 1992; 31: 14–21.

105. van Rooij LG, Toet MC, Osredkar D et al. Recovery of amplitude integrated electroencephalographic background patterns within 24 hours of perinatal asphyxia. Arch Dis Child Fetal Neonatal Ed 2005; 90: F245–51.

106. Holmes GL, Lombroso CT. Prognostic value of background patterns in the neonatal EEG. J Clin Neurophysiol 1990; 10: 323–52.

107. Azzopardi D, Guarino I, Brayshaw C et al. Prediction of neurological outcome after birth asphyxia from early continuous two-channel electroencephalography. Early Hum Dev 1999; 55: 113–23.

108. Biagioni E, Mercuri E, Rutherford M et al. Combined use of electroencephalogram and magnetic resonance imaging in full-term neonates with acute encephalopathy. Pediatrics 2001; 107: 461–8.

109. Toet MC, Hellström-Westas L, Groenendaal F, Eken P, de Vries LS. Amplitude integrated EEG at 3 and 6 hours after birth in fullterm neonates with hypoxic ischaemic encephalopathy. Arch Dis Child 1999; 81: F19–23.

110. Thornberg E, Ekström-Jodal B. Cerebral function monitoring: a method of predicting outcome in term neonates after severe perinatal asphyxia. Acta Paediatr 1994; 83: 596–601.

111. Eken P, Toet MC, Groenendaal F, de Vries LS. Predictive value of early neuromaging, pulsed Doppler and neurophysiology in full term infants with hypoxic–ischaemic encephalopathy. Arch Dis Child 1995; 73: F75–80.

112. Hellström-Westas L, Rosén I, Svenningsen NW. Predictive value of early continuous amplitude integrated EEG recordings on outcome after severe birth asphyxia in full term infants. Arch Dis Child 1995; 72: F34–8.

113. Shalak LF, Laptook AR, Velaphi SC, Perlman JM. Amplitude-integrated electroencephalography coupled with an early neurologic examination enhances prediction of term infants at risk for persistent encephalopathy. Pediatrics 2003; 111: 351–7.

114. Wertheim D, Mercuri E, Faundez JC et al. Prognostic value of continuous electroencephalographic recording in full term infants with hypoxic ischaemic encephalopathy. Arch Dis Child 1995; 71: F97–102.

115. ter Horst HJ, Sommer C, Bergman KA et al. Prognostic significance of amplitude-integrated EEG during the first 72 hours after birth in severely asphyxiated neonates. Pediatr Res 2004; 55: 1026–33.

116. Spitzmiller RE, Phillips T, Meinzen-Derr J, Hoath SB. Amplitude-integrated EEG is useful in perdicting neurodevelopmental outcome in full-term infants with hypoxic–ischemic encephalopathy: a meta-analysis. J Child Neurol 2007; 22: 1069–78.

117. Shany E, Goldstein E, Khvatskin S et al. Predictive value of amplitude-integrated electroencephalography pattern and voltage in asphyxiated term infants. Pediatr Neurol 2006; 35: 335–42.

118. Thorngren-Jerneck K, Hellström-Westas L, Ryding E, Rosén I. Cerebral glucose metabolism and early EEG/aEEG in term newborn infants with hypoxic- ischemic encephalopathy. Pediatr Res 2003; 54: 854–60.

119. Thornberg E, Thiringer K, Hagberg H, Kjellmer I. Neuron specific enolase in asphyxiated newborns: association with encephalopathy and cerebral function monitor trace. Arch Dis Child 1995; 72: F39–42.

120. Finer NN, Robertson CM, Richards RT, Pinnell LE, Peters KL. Hypoxic–ischemic encephalopathy in term neonates: perinatal factors and outcome. J Pediatr 1981; 98: 112–7.

121. Shah DK, Lavery S, Doyle LW et al. Use of 2-channel bedside electroencephalogram monitoring in term-born encephalopathic infants related to cerebral injury defined by magnetic resonance imaging. Pediatrics 2006; 118: 47–55.

122. Horan M, Azzopardi D, Edwards AD, Firmin RK, Field D. Lack of influence of mild hypothermia on amplitude-integrated-electroencephalography in neonates receiving extracorporeal membrane oxygenation. Early Hum Dev 2007; 83: 69–75.

123. Legido A, Clancy RR, Berman PH. Neurologic outcome after electroencephalographic proven neonatal seizures. Pediatrics 1991; 88: 583–96.

124. Mellits ED, Holden KR, Freeman JM. Neonatal seizures. II. A multivariate analysis of factors associated with outcome. Pediatrics 1982; 70: 177–85.

125. Robertson C, Finer N. Term infants with hypoxic–ischemic encephalopathy: outcome at 3.5 years. Dev Med Child Neurol 1985; 27: 473–84.

126. Menache CC, Bourgeois BF, Volpe JJ. Prognostic value of neonatal discontinuous EEG. Pediatr Neurol 2002; 27: 93–101.

127. Grigg-Damberger MM, Coker SB, Halsey CL, Anderson CL. Neonatal burst-suppression: its developmental significance. Pediatr Neurol 1989; 5: 84–92.

128. Steriade M, Amzica F, Contreras D. Cortical and thalamic cellular correlates of electroencephalographic burst-suppression. Electroencephalog Clin Neurophysiol 1994; 90: 1–16.

129. Aso K, Scher MS, Barmada MA. Neonatal electroencephalography and neuropathology. J Clin Neurophysiol 1989; 6: 103–23.

130. Aso K, Abdad-Barmada M, Scher MS. EEG and the neuropathology in premature neonates with intraventricular hemorrhage. J Clin Neurophysiol 1993; 10: 304–13.

131. Sherman DL, Brambrink AM, Ichord RN et al. Quantitative EEG during early recovery from hypoxic–ischemic injury in immature piglets: burst occurrence and duration. Clin Electroencephalogr 1999; 30: 175–83.

132. Osredkar D, Toet MC, van Rooij LGM et al. Sleep–wake cycling on amplitude-integrated EEG in full-term newborns with hypoxic–ischemic encephalopathy. Pediatrics 2005; 115: 327–32.

133. Toet MC, Lemmers PM, van Schelven LJ, van Bel F. Cerebral oxygenation and electrical activity after birth asphyxia: their relation to outcome. Pediatrics 2006; 117: 333–9.

134. Hahn JS, Vaucher Y, Bejar R, Coen RW. Electroencephalographic and neuroimaging findings in neonates undergoing extracorporeal membrane oxygenation. Neuropediatrics 1993; 24: 19–24.

135. Graziani LJ, Streletz LJ, Baumgart S, Cullen J, McKee LM. Predictive value of neonatal encephalograms before and during extracorporeal membrane oxygenation. J Pediatr 1994; 125: 969–75.

136. Pappas A, Shankaran S, Stockmann PT, Bara R. Changes in amplitude-integrated electroencephalography in neonates treated with extracorporeal membrane oxygenation: a pilot study. J Pediatr 2006; 148: 125–7.

137. Cowan F, Rutherford M, Groenendaal F et al. Origin and timing of brain lesions in term infants with neonatal encephalopathy. Lancet 2003; 361: 736–42.

138. Mercuri E, Rutherford M, Cowan F et al. Early prognostic indicators of outcome in infants with neonatal cerebral infarction: a clinical, electroencephalogram, and magnetic resonance imaging study. Pediatrics 1999; 103: 39–46.

139. de Vries LS, Toet MC. Amplitude integrated electroencephalography in the full-term newborn. Clin Perinatol 2006; 33: 619–32.

140. Papile L, Burstein L, Burstein R, Koffler H. Incidence and evolution of subependymal and intraventricular hemorrhage: a study of infants with birthweights less than 1500 g. J. Pediatr 1978; 92: 529–34.

141. Back SA. Perinatal white matter injury: the changing spectrum of pathology and emerging insights into pathogenetic mechanisms. MRDD Res Rev 2006; 12: 129–40.

142. Woodward LJ, Anderson PJ, Austin NC, Howard K, Inder TE. Neonatal MRI to predict neurodevelopmental outcomes in preterm infants. N Engl J Med 2006; 355: 685–94.

143. Watanabe K, Hakamada S, Kuroyanagi M, Yamazaki T, Takeuchi T. Electroencephalographical study of intraventricular hemorrhage in the preterm infant. Neuropediatrics 1983; 14: 225–30.

144. Radvanyi-Bouvet MF, de Bethmann O, Monset-Couchard M, Fazzi E. Cerebral lesions in early prematurity: EEG prognostic value in the neonatal period. Brian Dev 1987; 9: 399–405.

145. Clancy RR, Tharp BR, Enzman D. EEG in premature infants with intraventricular hemorrhage. Neurology 1984; 34: 583–90.

146. Connell J, Oozeer R, Regev R et al. Continuous four-channel EEG monitoring in the evaluation of echodense ultrasound lesions and cystic leucomalacia. Arch Dis Child 1987; 62: 1019–24.

147. Biagioni E, Bartalena L, Biver P, Pieri R, Cioni G. Electroencephalographic dysmaturity in preterm infants: a prognostic tool in the early postnatal period. Neuropediatrics 1996; 27: 311–16.

148. Hayakawa F, Okumura A, Kato T, Kuno K, Watanabe K. Dysmature EEG pattern in EEGs of preterm infants with cognitive impairment: maturation arrest caused by prolonged mild CNS depression. Brain Dev 1997; 19: 122–5.

149. Marret S, Parain D, Ménard J-F et al. Prognostic value of neonatal electroencephalography in premature newborns less than 33 weeks gestational age. Electroencephalogr Clin Neurophsysiol 1997; 102: 178–85.

150. Maruyama K, Okumura A, Hayakawa F et al. Prognostic value of EEG depression in preterm infants for later development of cerebral palsy. Neuropediatrics 2002; 33: 133–7.

151. Scher MS, Steppe DA, Banks DL. Prediction of lower developmental performances of healthy neonates by neonatal EEG-sleep measures. Pediatr Neurol 1996; 14: 137–44.

152. Saukkonen AL. Electroencephalographic findings in hydrocephalic children prior to initial shunting. Childs Nerv Syst 1988; 4: 339–43.

153. Al-Sulaiman AA, Ismail HM. Pattern of electroencephalographic abnormalities in children with hydrocephalus: a study of 68 patients. Childs Nerv Syst 1998; 14: 124–6.

154. Olischar M, Klebermass K, Kuhle S et al. Progressive posthemorrhagic hydrocephalus leads to changes of amplitude-integrated EEG activity in preterm infants. Childs Nerv Syst 2004; 20: 41–5.

155. Särkelä M, Mustola S, Seppänen T et al. Automatic analysis and monitoring of burst suppression in anesthesia. J Clin Monit Comput 2002; 17: 125–34.

156. Gürses D, Kiliç I, Sahiner T. Effects of hyperbilirubinemia on cerebrocortical electrical activity in newborns. Pediatr Res 2002; 52: 125–30.

157. Benders MJ, Meinesz JH, van Bel F, van de Bor M. Changes in electrocortical brain activity during exchange transfusions in newborn infants. Biol Neonate 2000; 78: 17–21.

158. Tallroth G, Lindgren M, Stenberg G, Rosen I, Agardh CD. Neurophysiological changes during insulin-induced hypoglycaemia and in the recovery period following glucose infusion in type 1 (insulin-dependent) diabetes mellitus in normal man. Diabetologia 1990; 33: 319–23.

159. Stenninger E, Eriksson E, Stigfur A, Schollin J, Aman J. Monitoring of early postnatal glucose homeostasis and cerebral function in newborn infants of diabetic mothers. A pilot study. Early Hum Dev 2001; 62: 23–32.

160. Theda C, Aygün C, Toet M et al. Amplitude-integrated EEG monitoring in patients with metabolic disorders. Abstract submitted to The 3rd International Conference on Brain Monitoring and Neuroprotection in the Newborn.

161. Markand ON, Garg BP, Brandt IK. Non-ketotic hyperglycinemia: electroencephalographic and evoked potential abnormalities. Neurology 1982; 32: 151–6.

162. Holmqvist P, Polberger S. Neonatal non-ketotic hyperglycinemia (NKH). Diagnosis and management in two cases. Neuropediatrics 1985; 16: 191–3.

163. Ohtsuka Y, Ohno S, Oka E. Electroclinical characteristics of hemimegalencephaly. Pediatr Neurol 1999; 20: 390–3.

164. Yamatogi Y, Ohtahara S. Early-infantile epileptic encephalopathy with suppression-bursts, Ohtahara syndrome; its overview referring to our 16 cases. Brain Dev 2002; 24: 13–23.

165. Hellström-Westas L, Blennow G, Rosén I. Amplitude integrated EEG (aEEG) in pyridoxine-dependent seizures and pyridoxine-responsive seizures. Acta Paediatr 2002; 91: 977–80.

166. Mikati MA, Trevathan E, Krishnamoorthy KS, Lombroso CT. Pyridoxine-dependent epilepsy: EEG investigations and long-term follow-up. Electrocencephalogr Clin Neurophysiol 1991; 78: 215–21.

167. Nabbout R, Soufflet C, Plouin P, Dulac O. Pyridoxine dependent epilepsy: a suggestive electroclinical pattern. Arch Dis Child Fetal Neonatal Ed 1999; 81: F125–9.

168. Klinger G, Chin CN, Otsubo H, Beyene J, Perlman M. Prognostic value of EEG in neonatal bacterial meningitis. Pediatr Neurol 2001; 24: 28–31.

169. Mikati MA, Feraru E, Krishnamoorthy K, Lombroso CT. Neonatal herpes simplex meningoencephalitis: EEG investigations and clinical correlates. Neurology 1990; 40: 1433–7.

183

Index

active sleep 18, 23
aEEG 2–3, 6–8, 36
  active sleep 23
  artifacts 9
  background patterns 19, 34–35
  classification 18–19, 34–35
  medication effects 19–21
    see also individual drugs
  monitors 10–11
  normal maturation 18, 26–29, 32–33
  perinatal asphyxia 79
  quiet sleep 30–31
  recovery after perinatal asphyxia 81, 86–87
  seizure patterns 61
  signal processing 2–3
  sleep-wake cycling 18, 21, 30–31
amplitude-integrated EEG *see* aEEG
anticonvulsant drugs 19–20, 83
  clonazepam 75, 136, 142, 164–165
  diazepam 20, 39
  fos-phenytoin
  lidocaine 20, 40, 97, 100, 136, 142, 162, 164
  midazolam 38, 74, 75, 97, 98, 100–101, 162, 166, 168
  phenobarbital
  phenytoin 20
  pyridoxine
artifacts 9, 43–56
  caregiving 48, 49, 80–81, 95, 97, 172
  electrode and head positioning 43, 51, 54–55
  electrocardiogram (ECG) 44, 56, 68
  gasping, hiccups 50, 89
  high-frequency ventilation 44, 53
  interelectrode distance 52
  loose electrode 45, 47
  muscle activity 46–47, 54–55

background patterns 19, 34–35
benign familial neonatal seizures 77–78

birth asphyxia 15, 63, 79–108
  hypothermia 79–80, 88–91
  hypoxic-ischemic encephalopathy 37, 57, 79
  prediction of outcome 80–81
  preterm infants 105–106
  recovery of aEEG background 81, 86–87
  seizures 80–81
  sleep-wake cycling 81–83
brain injury in preterm infants
  acute stage abnormalities 3, 12, 127
  aEEG/EEG continuity 127
  chronic stage abnormalities 3, 12, 127–128
  prediction of outcome 128–129
  seizures 128
  white matter damage 130–131
brain malformation 147–175
burst-suppression 19, 34–35, 81, 147

cerebellar hemorrhage 139–141
congenital heart disease 58, 62
continuous activity 19, 25, 34–35
continuous low voltage activity 19
cystic periventricular leukomalacia 127

density spectral array 60, 65
diazepam 20, 39
discontinuous activity 19, 34–35

EEG 1– 3, 5, 12, 17–25, 36
  neuronal basis for 1–2
  normal maturation 17–18, 23–25
  sleep-wake cycling 18, 21, 30–31
electroclinical 'uncoupling' 58, 63, 74–76
electrodes 2
electroencephalogram *see* EEG
extracorporeal membrane oxygenation (ECMO) 80

fentanyl 20
fifth-day seizures 57

gasping 50
germinal matrix/intraventricular hemorrhage 127

hemiconvulsions 109
hemimegalencephaly 147, 170–171
hemorrhagic lesions 127–146
    cerebellar hemorrhage 139–141
    GM-IVH 127
    intraparenchymal hemorrhage 116–117
    intraventricular hemorrhage 10, 22, 74–76
        full-term infant 116–117
        preterm infant 142–144
    thalamic hemorrhage 142–144
herpes simplex meningoencephalitis 147
high-frequency ventilation 53
hydrocephalus 31, 145
hypoglycemia 13, 57, 68–73, 147, 149–151
hypothermia 59, 88–91
hypoxia-ischemia 79–108
    hypothermia 79–80, 88–91
    perinatal asphyxia 79
    postasphyctic seizures 80
    reactivity to care 80–81
    recovery of aEEG background 81, 86–87
    sleep-wake cycling 81
hypoxic-ischemic encephalopathy 37, 57, 79

interburst interval (IBI) 14, 17–18, 25, 41, 49, 129
International 10-20 system 5
inactive background 19, 34–35, 86, 104–105, 107
incontinentia pigmenti 168–169
insulinoma 149–151
intracranial tumor 175
intraparenchymal hemorrhage 116–117, 136–138,
    121–124
intraventricular hemorrhage 10, 22, 74–76, 127–128,
    132–133
    full-term infant 116–117
    preterm infant 132–135, 139–144
ischemic lesions 127–146

lidocaine 20, 40, 97, 100, 136, 142, 162, 164
long-chain fatty acid disorder 152–154

medication effects 19–21
    see also individual drugs
meningitis 57, 162–167
    group B streptococcus 162–163
    bacillus cereus 164–165
    herpes simplex 147
    parechovirus 166–167
    respiratory syncytial virus 64
meningoencephalitis, see meningitis
metabolic diseases 147–161
    see also individual conditions
midazolam 20, 38, 74, 75, 97, 98, 100, 101, 162,
    166, 168

middle cerebral artery infarction 18, 110–115
    background asymmetry 110–113, 125–126
morphine 20, 39, 41
movement artifacts 43
muscle activity 47, 54–55

near-infrared spectroscopy 82
non-ketotic hyperglycinemia 147, 156–157

Ohtahara syndrome 147, 174
Ornithine transcarbamylase deficiency 155

perinatal asphyxia see birth asphyxia
periodic lateralized epileptiform discharges (PLED) 58
phenobarbitone 20, 37, 38, 75, 84, 100, 137, 142, 162,
    164, 168
pneumothorax 130–131
positive rolandic sharp waves 12, 18
posthemorrhagic ventricular dilatation 145
postconceptional age (PCA) 17
postmenstrual age (PMA) 17
postnatal age (PNA) 17
postoperative seizures 62
preterm infant
    acute stage abnormalities 127
    chronic stage abnormalities 127–128
    GMH-IVH 127, 132, 134–135
    IBI 18, 25
    intraparenchymal hemorrhage 116–117,
        136–137
    intraventricular hemorrhage 127, 132, 142–144
    ischemic lesions 127–146
    prediction of outcome 128–129
    seizures 128
    thalamic hemorrhage 142–144
    white matter damage 127, 130–131
pyridoxine-dependent seizures 57, 66–67, 147,
    158–159
pyridoxine-responsive seizures 158–159

quiet sleep 18, 24, 30

SAT (spontaneous activity transient) 17
secondary energy failure 92–96
sedatives 19–20, 38, 39
seizures 8, 9, 10, 12, 15, 48, 57–78
    benign familial neonatal 77–78
    congenital heart disease 62
    diagnosis
        automated detection 59–60
        clinical 58
        electrographic 58–59
    fifth-day seizures 57
    GMH-IVH 132–133
    incontinentia pigmenti 168–169
    meningitis 162
    postoperative 62

preterm infants 128
prognosis 60
pyridoxine 57, 66–67
sepsis 57
sleep
  active 23
  quiet 30
sleep-wake cycling 11, 18, 81
  classification of 19
  time at onset 83
spectrogram 15
spontaneous activity transients (SATs) 1
status epilepticus 10, 15, 37, 40, 61
  electroclinical uncoupling 58, 63, 74–76
  perinatal asphyxia 63
  subclinical 64, 68–71
  see also seizures

subdural hematoma 125–126
surfactant 20, 42

temporal sharp waves 18
thalamic hemorrhage 142–144
thalamocortical neurons 1, 5
tracé alternant 18, 19, 24, 29
tracé discontinu 15, 17, 24, 29
tuberous sclerosis 172–173

vein of Galen malformation 56

wakefulness 23, 30
watershed infarction 118–119
white matter injury 127, 130–131

Zellweger syndrome 160–161